I0024792

DANCING WITH GODDESSES

DANCING WITH GODDESSES
Archetypal Journey Through the Menstrual Cycle

by
Agnieszka Drabek-Prime

AEON

First published in 2025 by
Aeon Books

Copyright © 2025 by Agnieszka Drabek-Prime

The right of Agnieszka Drabek-Prime to be identified as the author of this work has been asserted in accordance with §§ 77 and 78 of the Copyright Design and Patents Act 1988.

All rights reserved. No part of this publication may be reproduced, stored in a retrieval system, or transmitted, in any form or by any means, electronic, mechanical, photocopying, recording, or otherwise, without the prior written permission of the publisher.

British Library Cataloguing in Publication Data

A C.I.P. for this book is available from the British Library

ISBN-13: 978-1-80152-163-5

Typeset by Medlar Publishing Solutions Pvt Ltd, India

www.aeonbooks.co.uk

A woman is born and grows, matures, gives birth to and nurtures all those around her. She grows old and dies. She is a circle within circle, a cycle within cycle, never ending, infinite. When women awaken and realize they have the ability to heal themselves, to impact their surroundings, they understand that they can change the order and laws of the world as we know it. When women learn themselves and their power and reclaim their strengths and potency, they can bring about global healing.

—Racheli Varulker

CONTENTS

PART 4: ENCHANTRESS—THE POWER OF THE SHAPESHIFTER

PART 5: WISE WOMAN AND THE WISDOM REGAINED

FOREWORD

Welcome fellow traveller on the path of the women's mysteries. Welcome to the journey of self-discovery and self-love. This is not an easy road. This trail is filled with questions, the unknown and often pain. But it is so worth pursuing as this is the way to the truth of who you are. This is the road to your inner-wisdom and beauty. This is the sacred spiral of life, death, and re-birth; the sacred spiral that you discover and follow every month with each new cycle. And with each cycle, you are being born anew, flow through the life given, die, and shed with your blood to be re-born again—wiser, stronger, and, if you allow it, each time more powerful. You have a choice to close your ears and your heart to the voice of your body and live pretending that it doesn't matter; or you can rise to the call and follow its path. There are no easy choices here. Whatever you decide to choose will bring its challenges. I have chosen to listen to my body and the wisdom of my blood, the wisdom of my cycle. I have chosen to be curious, to ask questions, and listen to the answers. I am a menstruating woman living in a male-oriented society. A society that has influenced my perception of myself, the world, and my place within it. This society offered me no guidance for the experiences of my menstrual cycle, nor for the feelings that arise from it. This society allowed me to believe that my cycle is a nuisance, not important, and that it stops my productivity and should be dealt with. This society allowed me to believe that my blood is shameful, dirty, and revolting. That my body and its amazing gifts were the sign of sin, and the presence of my menstrual cycle reinforced my inferior position in a male-dominated world. For a long time, I believed it to be true. In Western culture, which likes to think of itself as 'enlightened', the menstrual cycle is still rarely talked about or mentioned, unless in medical circumstances. There is such a profound feeling of shame associated with it that even mothers don't find it easy to introduce their daughters to the concept. It creates barriers and divisions not only between mothers and daughters, and women in general, but also the barrier between male and female deepens profoundly. Many women go through life hating themselves for cyclical feelings of irritability, tiredness, and depression. For many the experience of *Menarche* (the first period) was so traumatic they are still carrying it through their lives without the chance to talk about it, to process it, to welcome it. In our society the rites of passage have lost their meaning, and many women never feel welcomed into womanhood and its beautiful cyclicity. There is a plethora of women suffering both mentally and physically, but the only help given is to fight the symptoms or suppress them altogether. And menstruation remains a taboo. In society with its linear views of life and time, women that are cyclical by nature can't find their real place. We have forgotten that we are a part of the greater rhythms of the universe, and through our cyclical nature we can connect to these rhythms and gain wisdom and understanding. In times past, menstruation was considered holy. It was a sacred time when women could commune with the divine and channel the wisdom needed for the survival of their tribe. Women became the oracles for the greater good of all and for themselves. However, patriarchal cultures came to see it as a most dangerous time and created taboos around it. In Christianity, menstruation represents the original sin of Eve, a sin that is passed from mother to daughter; a sin that is very difficult to atone for. For a long time, both history (his-story) and society shaped our attitudes towards our bodies and menstruation. The time has come to take a fresh look and approach menstruation and our cyclicity anew. It is time to find out what it means to each individual woman. To discover the energies of our cycle—creativity and destruction—and find balance and harmony within our own natures using those energies for the good of ourselves, our communities, and the planet.

Therefore, I have decided to write this book. There are different ways you can work with your menstrual cycle. This is what I teach at my women's groups—how to be *Yoni* Wise. But for the purposes of this book, I would like to show you how you can discover the archetypes of the great goddesses and work with them to unravel the energy and feelings of your own cycle. There are so many lessons and stories in mythology that can answer many of our questions today. There are so many lessons in legends that can raise new questions. Questions that we as women must ask ourselves and pass on to our daughters. There is a thread, a weaving that we must follow to rediscover our importance, resources, and power. So please, take hold of the thread I am giving you. I have walked this path before you, so allow me to be your guide. Allow me to initiate you into the most important mysteries of your life: into the wisdom of your menstrual cycle; into your sacred spiral. Are you ready to begin? Take a deep breath in, hold on to the thread, and take your first step.

With love,
Agnieszka

INTRODUCTION

The healthy menstrual cycle

Let me tell you the story of your menstrual cycle. Before a woman is born her total supply of ovum is already contained in her ovaries. Her ability to mature and release these eggs begins during puberty and ends with the cessation of the menstrual cycle at menopause. The menstrual cycle is a beautiful weaving together that happens between the hypothalamus, pituitary glands, ovaries, and endometrium.

The onset of the first menstruation (*Menarche*) typically occurs between the ages of 10 and 16 years old. A woman will experience from 300–400 menstrual cycles in her lifetime. Menstrual bleeding lasts from 3–6 days in most women. Normal blood loss is considered to be 30–80 ml, and small clots are considered normal. The duration and amount of bleeding decline slightly in women over 35. However, women approaching menopause often experience significantly heavier bleeding than younger women.

For most girls, their first menstruation starts at around the age of 12 and this becomes known as the beginning of her cycle. The healthy menstrual cycle can last anything between 25–34 days. This cycle will become a very important part of a woman's life. Each month a woman's body undergoes a series of changes—variation in hormone balance, temperature, vaginal discharge, body weight, water retention, concentration levels, pain threshold, tiredness, and libido increase or decrease. It is imperative for each woman to become aware of how her body reacts and changes within her own cycle if she is to deepen her understanding of her own energy, creativity, and personality. Your monthly physical cycle consists of a few phases: menstrual, post-menstrual, pre-ovulatory, ovulatory, post-ovulatory, and pre-menstrual. The first day of your bleeding indicates the first day of your cycle. What marvels are beginning their dance in your body? When your bleeding ends, a miracle of creation takes place. By day 6 of your cycle, one of your ovaries will be readying itself for the egg release. Two hormones—follicle-stimulating hormone (FSH) and luteinising hormone (LH)—stimulate the follicle to increase oestrogen production. Your body is getting ready. There is a small elevation of progesterone a day or two before ovulation. Immediately before ovulation there is high oestrogen and the release of gonadotropin release hormone (GnRH) which suppresses FSH (the ovary is ready for release, and doesn't need any more stimulating). High oestrogen levels and a surge of LH from the anterior pituitary lead to ovulation, while the endometrium lining in your womb increases in thickness. Then rupture of the swollen follicle happens on approximately day 14 of the cycle, and with release of the ovum you are ovulating. The ovum can survive up to 72 hours after release, but it becomes less able to be fertilised after 35 hours. Higher secretion of progesterone raises your body temperature. Upon rapture of the follicle the cavity that held the ovum collapses and becomes blood-filled. This small amount of bleeding can cause irritation and lower abdominal pain of short duration during or straight after the ovulation. The blood is soon replaced with yellowish lipid-rich cells, forming corpus luteum (CL). After ovulation, the effects of the oestrogen and progesterone released by corpus luteum cause increased endometrial vascularisation and swelling. The secretory phase is designed to ready the uterus for implantation and pregnancy. Should conception occur, the corpus luteum persists and menstruation is inhibited until after the birth. Corpus luteum produces progesterone and oestrogen for one trimester of pregnancy and then this will be replaced by the placenta. Without conception, corpus luteum secretes oestrogen and progesterone with a peak in the middle of the luteal phase (day 23 of a 28-day cycle), then it begins to disintegrate about four days before the next *menses* (around day 24), when it is replaced by fibrous tissue forming corpus albicans. Baseline levels of oestrogen and progesterone trigger the hypothalamus to release GnRH which triggers the pituitary release of the FSH and the start of the new ovarian cycle. And then all the phases—menstruation, the follicular phase, ovulation, and the luteal phase—will carry on in a beautiful weave of cycles within your body. When you stop for a moment and think about what is happening within, you will discover this complicated and beautiful dance happening over and over again, with the perfection of the masterpiece that you are. And remember, before you are born your total supply of ovum is already contained in your ovaries. So please just think for a moment about this miracle. When you were in your mother's womb, the egg that would become your child was already within you. Contained with this beautiful possibility, generations within—*Yoni* within *Yoni*, life within life, cycle within cycle, into infinity. This is how the dance of the cycles began for you.

In the beautiful book *The Wise Wound* by Penelope Shuttle and Peter Redgrove, we read: 'every woman has ovaries as well as a womb, so what we call her menstrual cycle in fact consists of two cycles, ovarian and uterine, in interplay'. The ovarian cycle contains the ripening of the capsule containing the egg, ovulation, when the egg is released and captured by the Fallopian tube, and the last part when the remnants of the egg capsule create corpus luteum in preparation for pregnancy. The uterine cycle reflects the ovarian one. When oestrogen is being secreted by the ovary, the uterus responds by proliferating a new lining for itself after menstruation. At ovulation this suddenly stops, and a new phase starts, when the womb wall grows very thick in response to the secretion of the corpus luteum in the ovary. The womb lining develops deep glands that secrete a nutritive fluid that helps with egg implantation if it is fertilised. If it is not, then the ovarian secretion declines and without these hormones the new womb lining cannot sustain itself, 'its capillaries break up, and it is flushed out in the menstrual flow'. 'The ovary belongs to the species. It transmits the hereditary material'. A woman's womb is her own. Within this beautiful infinite dance, the wisdom of the species meets with the intimate inner-power of a woman. When it occurs consciously, miracles happen.

I love and appreciate my cycle and my period now, but I didn't feel like that at the beginning. I allowed myself to believe when I was told that not only my period was a nuisance, but also that suppressing it was a normal and healthy thing to do. I also believed that my cycle didn't matter unless I was trying to conceive. But the truth is that your menstrual cycle should be monitored as one of the vital signs.

> Once young females begin menstruating, evaluation of the menstrual cycle should be included with an assessment of other vital signs. By including this information with the other vital signs, clinicians emphasise the important role of menstrual patterns in reflecting overall health status.
>
> (American Academy of Pediatrics and American College of Obstetricians and Gynecologists, 'Menstruation in Girls and Adolescents: Using the Menstrual Cycle as a Vital Sign'. *Pediatrics*, 118 (5) (2006): 2248)

Observing and taming my cycle allowed me to notice things that weren't right within my body. That also helped me with the adenomyosis diagnosis and learning how to help myself live with this condition. It also allowed me to understand myself so much better—everything that was happening to me and my body, my emotions, thoughts, all the cyclical blessings and anathemas, blisses, and pains. And it may be surprising for you to know that although common in belief, moderate to severe pain with menstruation is not normal or healthy. Pain is a sign that something is wrong. Unfortunately, we have many centuries of minimising the experiences of women and female bodies as a whole. I can understand that monthly pain making you feel like you are dying is not likely to make you love your menstrual cycle. I know, I have been there and oftentimes still am (thanks to adenomyosis flare-ups). But tracking my cycle helped me to understand where I was and what was happening. It also helped me to put healthy self-care measures in place. It's not always easy—it's life and life rarely is. But your menstrual cycle is your vital sign. The sign of overall health of your body and mind. A sign that is responding to everything that is happening in your life. I would like to encourage you to take up the role of a witness and observer, and with love and compassion monitor your cycle. Record what you can see, without judgement or jumping to any conclusions. Your menstrual cycle is simply responding to your environment. It is simply responding to you. Your menstrual cycle contains great wisdom and power. Your cycle is part of a greater whole, a universal energy that is propelling you towards becoming the most vibrant and authentic version of yourself. It allows you to discover your sexual energy, and sexual energy is creative by its very nature. It allows you to create your reality and create your masterpieces day by day. How long have you been ignoring your body? If your periods are too painful to bear, there is a reason for that. Your body is trying to communicate with you. Bodies talk to us in a very subtle way, but if we keep ignoring them, they will shout at us to listen. Your body shouts in pain. Maybe it is time to start to pay attention. With each period you are shedding the energy of the cycle past and venture into a new journey. Your cycle has a natural flow allowing you to feel more energised and vibrant at certain times and more withdrawn at others. It's time to embrace your cyclical nature and the gifts it brings to you. With each menstrual cycle comes the opportunity to know yourself better, to connect with your inner-wisdom and step into your feminine power. Your cycle is a piece of the universal puzzle. As women, we are part of the greater cycle within cycle and we have the ability to not only observe them, but also understand ourselves, our power and the universal web of life.

Cycle within cycle

The idea behind the Medicine Wheel has a very significant importance in my life. Originally it was received by cultures living closely with the Earth and Nature. Most of us learnt about the Medicine Wheel from Native American culture, but it was also present in the Slavic countries and in Druidic Britain. It is a living map of empowerment given from the Earth to all of us. It is a circular system that never ends and is both teaching us and learning from us. In the Medicine Wheel, a few layers build upon each other. In the first instance, we have a basic wheel which gives us four directions—East, South, West, and North. Each direction will carry a corresponding element—East and Air, South and Fire, West and Water, North and Earth. In different traditions, the correspondences between directions and elements may be different. To complete the wheel, we would add Great Above, Great Below and Great Within. The wheel is in constant movement following the movement of planets, and of our lives—the movement of creation. It is a map that is very much alive and we as women are the embodiment of that map. There are many circles and cycles within the Medicine Wheel. They are the global cycles of creation, but also our personal, individual cycles.

The moon wheel

The moon cycle lasts 28 days, just as the average menstrual cycle does. Within the moon cycle, we can observe a new moon, waxing moon, full moon, waning moon, dark moon and then the beginning of the new cycle with the next new moon. Within the energy of the moon cycle, we can notice the rise, peak and waning of the energy. Exactly what we can observe within our menstrual cycle. We witness 13 moons per solar year, and as women we are dying and being re-born 13 times each year. Women are lunar creatures. In many languages words describing the moon will be used to describe menstruation as well: moon-time or *miesiączka* (Polish, from the month, *miesiąc* and the moon). The moon itself will be identified with the lunar goddess, or in languages where the word 'moon' holds masculine gender (like for example in Polish we have *ten księżyc*)—the moon will be the master of women. Looking at the moon and menstruation, we can clearly see the resemblance.

– Dark moon—the void.
– New moon—new cycle/menstruation/bleed.
– Waxing moon—post-menstrual and pre-ovulation.
– Full moon—ovulation.
– Waning moon—post-ovulation and pre-menstrual.
– And then the dark moon again.

In this way, the phases of the moon mirror our personal journey through our individual Medicine Wheel, becoming another cycle within the previous cycle and adding another wheel to the medicine of the universe.

The sun wheel

The journey that the bright sun takes across the sky also reflects the personal journey of our women's mystery. Within the sun wheel, we can observe the inner sun wheel, which is the sun's daily voyage:

– Night—menstruation (with the void at midnight).
– Dawn—post-menstrual.
– Midmorning—pre-ovulation.

– Noon—ovulation.
– Afternoon—post-ovulation.
– Dusk—pre-menstrual.
– And then night again.

But we can also observe the outer sun wheel that will take us through the seasons.

– Winter—pre-menstrual and Menstruation.
– Spring—post-menstruation and pre-ovulation.
– Summer—parts of pre-ovulation and ovulation.
– Autumn—post-ovulation and part of pre-menstrual.

The beautiful sun adds a third level to our medicine with the wheel of tropical seasons. The tropical seasons reflect our cervical juices and mucus production.

– Cool and dry—winter.
– Dry—spring.
– Hot and sticky—summer.
– Rainy—autumn.

The wheel of life

This is a cosmic wheel of creation. Everything in the universe flows through that wheel.

Birth–childhood–adulthood–elderhood–death–?
Can you see the correlation to your menstrual cycle here as well?

The archetypal wheel

Every month our menstrual cycle takes us on a different journey and each phase of our cycle will call forth a different archetype. This is what this book is all about. How we can work with different archetypes to get to know ourselves better, to understand ourselves, and to know where we are in the present moment on our Medicine Wheel.

– Menstruation—Dark Goddess.
– Post-menstrual—Maiden.

– Pre-ovulation—Lover.
– Ovulation—Mother.
– Post-ovulation—Enchantress.
– Pre-menstrual—Sage/Crone.

The Medicine Wheel is not set in stone. It is a living map that can differ from woman to woman. What is important to remember is that our menstrual cycle circles through our psyche each month, taking us through different aspects of ourselves. Within the Medicine Wheel, time and space doesn't exist. The wheel takes us from our present to our past and can visit our future before coming back to the present once more. If we struggle through a certain phase of our menstrual cycle, it is always worth going back to what happened to us during the corresponding time in our lives. If your menstruation is painful and you struggle badly even though physically everything is great, it is important to revisit the Maiden part of your Wheel of Life. What is hiding in your psyche— was there a sexual assault, a trauma, an accident that re-plays itself in your soul month after month, cycle after cycle? By working with that past trauma, you can improve and heal your present. Therefore, understanding our cyclicity is crucial in healing ourselves and our society. It is also important to remember that we are not running in circles like headless chickens. Our journey is the Spiral Path. Although we are travelling through our Medicine Wheel, through the archetypes repeatedly, we are never coming back to the same place. Through our Wheel of Life, we are constantly changing, maturing, and growing and because of that each of our maidens will be different, each of our menstruations will be different, because we are approaching it from a different place on our wheel. And this is how cycles within cycles turn and propel us to dive deeper into our feminine mysteries. Kind of the same, but every time different, spiralling again and again, rising, peaking, and waning with our personal energy and the energy of the universe.

Cycle tracking

Our cycle is one of our vital signs and I cannot stress enough the importance of cycle tracking. Being curious and paying attention are the first steps. Following them will lead you to what Lisa Hendrickson-Jack called 'body literacy'. This literacy will uncover not only moments of your fertility, but also will reveal general changes your body is going through each month, and will help you to track the changes in your health. Cycle tracking was my main tool in discovering patterns that led to my adenomyosis diagnosis. Cycle tracking allows me to see where I am, and what is happening physically, emotionally, and energetically within my body. It also allows me to plan my activities and workload. It explains to me certain behaviours or feelings I may notice. For example, knowing that I'm feeling down on certain days is due to the transition in my cycle, helps me to relax into those feelings, finding compassion and kindness for myself. Cycle tracking taught me also that nothing is stuck in time. Everything is in constant movement. Our emotions, feelings, and fears are in constant movement as well, they're not static—even if sometimes it would seem so. I know now that everything will pass, whatever I am feeling and experiencing in this moment will pass as well. Regardless of whether this feeling is pleasant or terrifying. The wisdom of the cycle translates itself into life wisdom I can draw from every day. It also helps me to understand and relate to other women. To understand their changes and flows. And by checking and sharing with each other where in our cycle we are, we can truly arm ourselves in compassion and love, and see one another as equals, not taking things personally all the time. We are sisters in our cyclicity and understanding that can only bring us closer. Finding a tribe of like-minded women was the best thing that has happened to me. Being seen, accepted, and understood for where we are in our cycle brings a different level to our friendships and human interactions. We can cycle track as a means to track our fertility when we are trying to conceive or avoiding pregnancy altogether. But we should also cycle track to get to know ourselves, our feelings, and our energy patterns. Cycle tracking will make us intimate with our *Yoni*, which is the power centre for every woman. This book is not a guide to fertility awareness or how to avoid pregnancy; it is more of a journey of self-discovery. Spending time each day connecting to your womb, by dropping down into your body with curiosity and open heart will allow you to become intimate with yourself, maybe even for the first time in your life. We are raised to give our intimacy to others, but self-intimacy is harder to come by. Yet, it is one of the most important gifts we can present to ourselves. It is not a chore, we have too many of those already. It is a self-care practice, so please approach it as such.

How to track your cycle

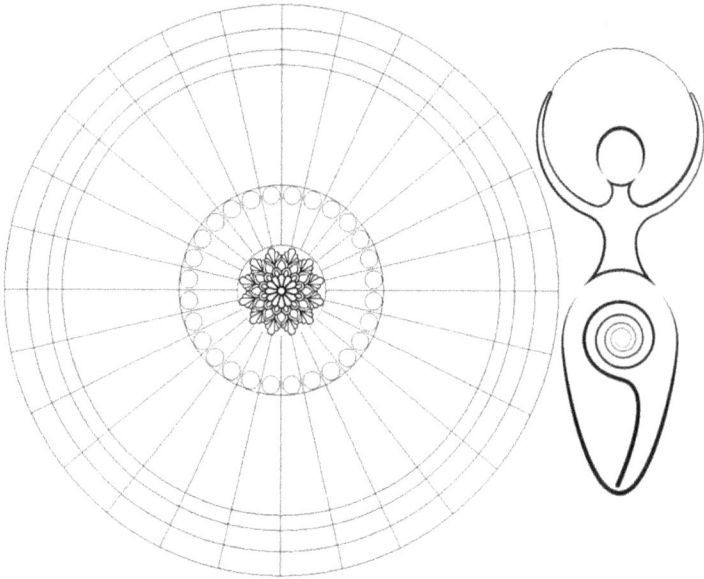

Medicine wheel of 28 day cycle

Here I am offering you a beautiful cycle tracker designed by my beautiful friend, Diana Gavazzo. The pdf version can be downloaded from my website, www.primetherapy.co.uk (please look at the 'Yoni Wise' section of the site). You can make it your own by colouring it differently for each cycle. The goddess is holding an orb in which you can place the intention or the motto for this cycle, something you would like to work on through that cycle, a quote that has inspired you, or a message from your womb that you may have received during your meditation. The first day of your cycle is the first day of your menstruation. So, each time you start a new menstruation, you will start a new cycle tracker as well. On the outer circle of your tracker write the day of your cycle—from 1 to 28 or however long your cycle is. In the middle circle you can colour-code your mood, and in the last circle put today's date. After that, you will have a space for the message from your womb, or for a description of how you are feeling on that day. To be perfectly honest, you can write there whatever your heart/womb desires. This is your space of self-discovery. If like me you like journaling, this space is not nearly enough, so carry on writing in your journal. This is your starting point and putting together cycle trackers from a few months will help you to see what your cycle looks like, what days are harder, whether they occur cyclically or not, when you are ovulating, and how regular your cycle is. In the little circle near the middle, you have space to indicate what is happening with the moon on that day. I've mentioned already how important the moon is for us women. Putting your cycle phase in relation to the moon phase will allow you to go much deeper. It may also explain certain behaviours or feelings. Do you remember when we were talking earlier about moon cycles and we put ovulation together with a full moon? I personally prefer to ovulate during or near the dark moon and menstruate during the full moon. When I'm ovulating, my energy is often too much for me to bear and when added to the mix the energy of the full moon, well let's just say I find it challenging. But when I ovulate during a dark moon, I can feel my energy being drawn back by the moon, which helps me to stay focused and grounded. At the same time when I'm menstruating during the full moon, I feel myself held up by the energy of the moon and that prevents me from diving deeply into the abyss. Also depending on the moon phase, which may be waxing or waning, we will be under the influence of rising or falling energy—expansion or contraction. Please give it a go and see how deeply you can travel within yourself. Let go of expectations and open yourself to curiosity and adventure. Allow yourself to meet the real you.

Womb meditation

I've learnt this way of meditating from Melanie Swan of *The Sacred Womb* and adapted it to reflect different phases and energies. It is a lovely way to connect to your womb, to drop in and check how you truly are today. Without putting on false appearances, without expectation, just dropping deeply into the core of your being. Into the place that holds the wisdom of who you are. From this place, you can weave your truth. From this place, you can see all. From this place, you just *know*. The womb is where our power resides. It is awakened during *Menarche*—our first bleed, then takes us on a journey of discovery throughout our bleeding years, and deepens during the menopause—when we become Elders, Wise Women. The womb is a portal, a place of weaving, of creation. From this place, we give birth to our human children, but also to our idea-children. This is the place of happening, of conjuring; this is the centre of our individual universe. By daily dropping in, you can become truly intimate with yourself, and you can begin to know yourself on a different level. The understanding that you will unravel will allow you to find happiness with who you are. Because you are perfect already, you have just forgotten that for a moment. If for any reason you no longer have a physical womb, please don't worry. Your energetic and spiritual wombs are still there. Your womb space is ready to welcome you and heal the trauma of removed organs, of pain and fear. Trust your body, trust your energy, trust the universe. This meditation is for all of us. This healing is for all of us.

To connect to your womb, sit or lay down comfortably with your hands on your lap or by the side of your body if you have chosen to lie down. Breathe easily and gently—in through your nose and out through your nose or mouth—you choose. How would you like to breathe today? Notice the cold air coming in through your nose, the air is warming up inside of your body and then the warm air is coming out of your mouth (or nose). Breathe like that for a moment, in and out, gently, naturally. Notice that with each breath your breathing is becoming slower and deeper, and that with each breath your body is becoming more and more relaxed. Now I would like to invite you to begin the wave breath. On the in-breath take the energy and the breath from the bottom of your feet and allow it to travel up your body to the top of your head. On a gentle pause between in-breath and out-breath, allow this energy to linger at the top of your head, and then on the out-breath flow the energy and the breath down your body to your feet. In and up, out and down. Breathe like that for a few in-breaths and out-breaths. Now, if you are ready, please place your hands on your womb (the space between your belly button and your pubic bone). On the in-breath allow the breath and the energy to travel up to the top of your head, pause there for a second and on the out-breath allow it to slowly flow into your womb space. You can drop fast or float very slowly—depending on your day and on the phase of your cycle. How do you feel today? Are you ready to drop fast, or will you allow your breath to slowly seep within? Follow whatever is happening. This is your body and your practice. But whatever way you choose, drop deeply into your womb space. Breathe deeply in and out of your womb space. This is the space of your power, of your creativity, of your strength. Breathe deeply. Feel your womb welcoming you. *Welcome home, my darling*. You have arrived. Breathe deeply. Feel the warmth of your hands on your belly, feel the warmth of your breath within your womb. You are safe, you are grounded, you are loved. Look around. What does your womb look like today? How does she feel? Ask her for a message, for a colour. See what story she will gift you with today. Stay with yourself, with your womb. And if there is no colour, no message, that is absolutely fine. Just stay with what is, and what comes forth to the surface. No message is also the message. Rest and silence are equally important. Listen to the wisdom of your womb, and spend some time together. And when you are ready, thank your womb for your time together. Gather this beautiful energy and on the in-breath take it up to your heart space. On the out-breath drop it down to your womb again. On the in-breath to your heart—on the out-breath to your womb. We move this energy to our heart space, so we can feel our truth. Next time when you breathe in move this energy to your throat, and on the out-breath drop it back to your womb space. In and up to your throat, out and down to your womb. We bring this energy to our throat, so we can speak our truth. Next time you breathe in, please move this beautiful womb energy to the top of your head, and then back down to your womb on the out-breath. In and up to the top of your head. Out and down, back to your womb. We bring this energy to the top of our head, so we can know our truth. Next time when you breathe into the top of your head, pause there for a second and then on the out-breath allow this beautiful womb energy to flow all over you. Envelop yourself in this healing energy like in a cocoon. What colour does this energy present for you today? Feel yourself loved, safe, and grounded. Take a deep breath in and out and let go of this energy. Allow it to flow where it wants to, don't try to force it or push it in any direction. Let go, breathe naturally and slowly start to bring yourself back into your body. Introduce gentle movement and stretching and when you're ready, but only when you are ready, open your eyes.

How was your journey of self-discovery? Now that you have returned, take your cycle tracker and write all the information on it. What day of the cycle you are on today? What colour and message did your womb grant you? Where is the moon on her journey through the sky? Can you see yourself as a part of a greater whole? As part of universal weaving? Your cycle is intertwined with other cycles. They all inform each other, they feed each other and are fed in return, they inform each other and take back all the information they need. You are not separate. We are all connected. All around us, the universe is alive. We've been told that creation happened at the beginning of time, but it's not the entire truth, is it? Creation is happening every single minute. It happens within us and all around us. The cosmic web of life is in constant movement, constant flow. And so are we, an inevitable part of creation.

Why goddesses?

For a long time in his-story, the feminine was demonised. Our bodies were perceived as unclean and polluting to ourselves and others, and our souls as damned from the moment of our birth. If we look back to the story of Eve told from that perspective, we have a prime example of his-story of the first sin. Eve picked up the fruit and shared it with her man. She touched the Tree of Knowledge, which is also the Tree of Life. With this fruit, she chose the rhythms of nature, the knowledge of life, death, and re-birth, and the menstrual power to understand the flow of the universe. But this gift was seen as a symbol of betrayal. Eve was blamed for bringing death and evil into the world. From now on you will birth in pain—said the God. But how many children did Eve birth in Paradise painlessly? Bleeding Eve was thrown out of the Garden and mortal death took us into its possession. Death that was seen as an end rather than part of a continuing cycle. The curse went further, taking with it female sexuality and fertility. To this day menstruation is perceived and called 'the curse'. But in truth, what we know as a curse was in fact a gift. A gift of the cyclical nature of menstruation connecting us to the web of life. Connecting us to the rhythms of nature and of the universe. Allowing us to see the interconnectedness between ourselves and the cycles of life. It gives us hope that nothing is final, and that after death, there is a re-birth. We know it deeply in our bodies as we live through it month after month, cycle after cycle. We know one part of the story. But it's time to give voice to the other part. The hidden part of the feminine mysteries.

We communicate and understand the world through stories. Stories are our teachers; they provide a lens through which to find a meaningful way of explaining the laws of life. Archetypes are perfect examples of people and things, inherited from our earliest ancestors and still present in the collective unconscious, and still present in your subconsciousness. Our ancestors told the stories of strong and powerful goddesses. But those stories are still relevant now. They show divine beings through the eyes of ordinary women. They teach us how to reconnect to our feminine power, and how to find divinity within. How to find the wisdom that was thought of as long lost. Those teachings, the understanding, the messages, are still there for us to find and decipher. They are there so we can listen deeply with our inner ear, with our heart, and begin to weave a new story—her-story to balance his-story. So, we can become the heroines of our own journey. So, we can rediscover our bodies, our pleasure, and the feminine wisdom of our ancestors. So, we can listen. So, we can become. So, we can break the reign of the curse and accept it for the gift it really is. Stories are medicine, and we are powerful medicine women. The time is now.

How to work with this book?

As working with archetypes is very individual, please listen to your own heart. I'll guide you through a few archetypes for each phase of your menstrual cycle, but please choose only the ones that speak to you. You may feel drawn to certain parts of the work and not to others, and that is perfect. This is your journey and yours alone. If you are no longer bleeding, you may venture on a year-long journey through the goddess archetypes. Start from the section of the book that corresponds to the season you now find yourself in. You can also choose the moon as your guide and follow the archetypes in this way. If you are still bleeding, you can go on a year-long journey or you can choose to work through the archetypes according to your menstrual phase. Choose one for each phase and maybe then a different one for the next cycle. Again, this is your journey, and you are your own authority. The work can be devotional, if you choose so, or it can be simply the work with the archetypes, and stories to bring understanding and example. Each goddess will bring some exercises or meditations for you to try. Again, try them all, or only the ones you feel drawn to. If you find the exercises helpful—weave them into your routine, into the rhythm of your cycle. Create your own rituals and pass them on to your daughters, granddaughters, and nieces, and share them with your friends. Create a circle of like-minded women and practice them together, sharing your insights and experiences afterwards.

Remember, the more you sow the bigger your harvest will become. If you feel so inclined, create the altar for your journey. This will be your womb altar. I am a great believer in the power of manifestation through the altar. For each season (the inner one or the outer one) change the cloth on your altar and add some seasonal symbolism. If your work is devotional, add items that symbolise the goddess you are working with. If your work is not devotional, add items that symbolise the archetypes for you—strength, courage, flow, femininity. Each goddess will bring different messages. Listen to them and manifest them into reality through your altar and through your body. You can burn candles on your altar while meditating, or you can meditate while lying in your bed or sitting in a chair. Make this practice your own.

Please make journaling the key part of your practice. I can't stress enough the importance of putting your thoughts on paper. By documenting your experiences, feelings, and setbacks you will be able to gain a wider perspective of the process and of your own journey. Don't allow the belief that you will remember to stop you. You won't remember, that's how our memory works. But you can be reminded by your own words, and you can revisit your past and its medicine. By having a dedicated journal, you can also answer the questions posed to you in each phase. This is your journey, and you will be able to notice, understand, and learn from this process in order to heal. But there is one requirement. Your honesty to yourself and a commitment to your cycle.

For meditations, read them to yourself first and then try to follow them from memory, or if you prefer, record the meditations yourself and then listen to them through the headphones. For my personal practice, I often record meditations first and then replay them to myself when needed. You can also find some meditations on my website, so please go to www.primetherapy.co.uk, relax, and enjoy.

One more requirement before we begin. Track your cycle: like a hawk, circling from above focused on the smallest things; like a doe, finding a path even through the thickest undergrowth; like a turtle, flowing through the currents; like a dove, filled with hope and wonder; like a lioness, protecting her sovereignty and the sacredness of her body. Track your cycle daily: note, observe, discover. This is the key to your healing and to your growth. Track your cycle passionately. With love and compassion to your emotions and to your body. Track your cycle with curiosity. Track it with an open heart. Have a blessed journey!

PART 1

WINTERING IN MENSTRUAL WISDOM

CHAPTER 1

The wisdom of the void

Message from the void

I'm writing today from the depth of my void. From the place in between. From the place of wisdom and maturity of my cycle gone by. I'm filled with the wisdom of my blood. It spins and spirals within my womb nourishing my thoughts, feelings, and physical organs. Deep within I have answers to all my questions. Deep within lay the answers to all the questions asked by the world. All within my womb: closed; held. It is in my power to connect to that wisdom, or to let it go with the upcoming bleed without connecting, with no answers. The wisdom will soak into the earth and the mother will mature that knowledge within. I'm holding hands on my womb, and I can feel the pulse of life. Blood is life, even within the void and at this moment I am filled with my blood to the brim. All new ideas come to life through the pulsation of my womb, through my hands and then out, into the world. My hands, overcome with this inner-wisdom, are writing these words, from within, from the portal of my creativity. I feel pregnant and abundant with ideas, with life. I am able to create. I am the creatrix and I shape my entire world into being. As this fullness and the oneness bubble into the surface, I can also see the winter behind the void. The wintering is announced by the first drop of blood released from within. But before I open myself to this release, I'm allowing myself to delve deeply within my inner cauldron. I'm allowing myself to dive into the mystery of my own essence. Essence that is me. I—the wise one; I—the creatrix; I—the goddess suspended within the void of my being. And today my void is no darkness. It is filled with light, filled with brightness, and I can feel it radiating through my body. Today I am the light, I am the bright one. I can feel peace and calmness. I can feel the beauty within the heaviness of my breasts and the fullness of my hips. And I know this is not how the void always looks. But this is the gift of the void today. And I am cherishing this gift with an open heart and gratitude. I can feel my breath coming into my body and then gently leaving and I am able to see the light coming in and out as well. And with each breath, the particles of all are entering my body, and I am filled with the outside world—as within so without. And with each out-breath, I am giving myself out into the world, in sacred sharing and communion. The particles of me mixed with the particles of All. And I can feel so much happiness through this exchange. And as my body is becoming heavier and heavier, through entering my personal winter I know I will become lighter and lighter. I know because I listen within, to my inner needs, to the needs of my body. And as my body is lying here resting, my mind and spirit are soaring through the void, through the portal of my womb into infinity. And I know that by listening and acknowledging I can soar beyond infinity. So, I listen deeply, truly, with an open heart. I listen with my body as this is the wisdom too diffi-cult for my mind to comprehend. And as I listen, I become. And my 'I' merges with the 'All that is'. And I just *know*, deep down within my bones, within my womb—the primal knowledge never forgotten, but stored. And I am so grateful for this knowledge and for this medicine. I am so grateful for the teachings of my void. My blood will come soon and the energy of what I am experiencing right now will shift again. And I am not going to stop it. I wouldn't be able to even if I wanted to. I'm going to follow that spiral of my womanhood with trust and an open heart. But for now, I am immersing myself within the song of my void, within this primal call.

What message does your void sing for you? Close your eyes. Listen. Become.

What is the void

Please close your eyes, connect to your womb, and breathe deeply. From this place ask yourself and look for the answers within. What does the void mean to me? What pictures, messages, and insights does this word bring up? What your womb is showing and telling you?

I can tell you what it means to me.

To me, the void is both: a vast emptiness—the ending, but also a bright expanse—the beginning.

The void is a liminal place, the space in between. This is the moment when your old cycle has ended, but the blood hasn't flown yet and the new cycle hasn't yet begun. You are filled with your blood and your inner cauldron is bubbling with knowledge, insight, and power. This is the place where gods dwell and where you can meet and walk with the spirit/god/goddess.

It is the place of power, but power is not good or evil. It can be used for either this or that, but power itself just is. And so is the power in your womb. It is. Held in-between—between the maturity of your old cycle and the innocence of the new one. Between the death of the old cycle, and the birth of the new one. It is a place without expectations, a place of learning and self-discovery. But it is not always glorifying. Often this moment in your cycle is raw and painful. And as the cycle is translated into our lives, so is the void. And the voids in our lives can be both—places of expansion, growth, and insight, and terrifying, raw almost nightmares filled with pain and fear.

But the void is also the great emptiness. The suspension in between. In this place, you may feel nothing, or you may feel so much and that feeling will be so intense it will almost make you numb. The emptiness can have a twofold attribute. It can simply be just that, a place of emptiness, a suspension in timelessness, without roots and gravity—there is so much healing there. Or it may be a place to be filled with. In empty, there is so much space for the new—new discoveries, feelings, paths, new you. Your beautiful body will lead you there and your womb will become the portal of your transformation. Is it easy? No. Why? Because the void is the most vulnerable moment in the entire cycle. Our energy is at its lowest and often it feels as though the ground was taken out from underneath our feet. We may have been coping and managing till this moment all daily challenges and then, whoosh, we lose the thread.

We stand face to face with our naked truth—without any filters, any inhibitions and all the monsters seem to be coming out from all the dark places within. They are coming to the surface, and sometimes right out of us. The void moment can be a time of the deepest darkness. Sometimes the hole may become so deep it may feel like that's it—like destruction is the only way out. It can be a bleak place. However, when we stop fighting and try to open ourselves to it, the void can become the great unknown. A place of new potential and new possibility. It can become a mirror through which we can see our true face. If we allow this gap in the fabric of life to open, we may allow a spiritual connection to enter. We may see beyond what was and what is yet to come. We may become the oracles for our own lives. This moment of void is the most powerful place in the cycle. We can experience a profound feeling of union, we can shed and let go of our old ways, drop our masks, and look beyond allowing life to change us. Allowing ourselves to enter the flow of the liminal. And as the liminal place is not governed by time nor space, we can travel into places we've never been before. We can come into a new conversation with the spirit, with ourselves, with the world. We need to give ourselves this space to experience the void, to learn from it, to expand. We need to soften into this place, knowing it's coming. We need to dive deeply within the filled cauldron of our womb and stay there for as long as it takes to let go, for our flow to announce a new beginning, a new cycle, a return from timelessness into time and space. And in the wisdom of our withheld blood, we can look ourselves in the eye and find new medicine and answers to most questions.

The void in our cycle is that space just before the bleeding. It can last from a few minutes, through a few hours, to even 2–3 days. It's the place in between the old and new cycle. You can feel the old cycle has already finished, but the new cycle hasn't started yet. And if we allow the lessons from the void of our cycle in, it will help us immensely to travel through the void in our everyday lives. Life is also filled with the void—in a day, in a week, in a year, in the death and life of our loved ones. Void is an integral part of being alive, and we as women can become accomplished practitioners of travelling through it. Examples of voids in life cycles: dark moon (0% visibility), midnight, noon, between Christmas and New Year, between death and burial, there is a void in a moment of dying, at the top of each in-breath and out-breath, in the birthing room during transitions there is a void in each transition.

So next time when you find yourself faced with the void, don't run away, don't fight. Simply slow down, with curiosity, compassion and self-love and see what messages are flowing to you through this myste-rious place. And if it hurts, let it be so. And if it is overwhelming, let it be so. Just drop down into your womb space and trust.

The void meditation

Sit down comfortably. Breathe easily and gently—in through your nose and out through your nose or mouth—you choose. How would you like to breathe today? Notice the cold air coming in through your nose, the air is warming up inside of your body and then the warm air is coming out of your mouth (or nose). Breathe like that for a moment, in and out, gently, naturally. Notice that with each breath your breathing is becoming slower and deeper, and that with each breath your body is becoming more and more relaxed. Now I would like to invite you to begin the wave breath. On the in-breath take the energy and the breath from the bottom of your feet and allow it to travel up your body to the top of your head. On a gentle pause between in-breath and out-breath, allow this energy to linger at the top of your head, and then on the out-breath flow the energy and the breath down your body to your feet. In and up, out and down. Breathe like that for a few in-breaths and out-breaths. Now, if you are ready, please place your hands on your womb. On the in-breath allow the breath and the energy to travel up to the top of your head, pause there for a second and on the out-breath allow it to slowly flow into your womb space. Slowly and gently, through your throat, through your heart—your mighty drum, right down into your womb space. Take as much time as you need. Breathe deeply in and out of your womb space. Allow the life-giving force of your breath to enter your womb. Breathe fully into your womb space.

And as your attention is in your womb now, I would like to invite you to notice that she is very dark. Let this dark womb be like dark earth. You are allowed to become still, to become quiet. You are allowed to submerge yourself in the darkness. Notice any fears and resistance that come up from going into these depths of darkness. Notice them with gentleness and compassion towards yourself. You don't have to do anything with them, just notice and let go of any expectations. And if you are willing, also notice the comfort of being in this place, relaxation, freedom. Notice how you feel here.

Your womb is a portal to the depths of Mather Earth. Here you can see what is ready to sprout, to germinate. What is ready to show itself to you? But you can also notice here what is ready to die, what you are ready to let go of. And if you are ready and willing, let go of it, fully, filled with trust. Breathe deeply.

Life begins in the darkness, in the depths of the void. What is your gift growing in the darkness right now? What is your medicine for the coming weeks and months? Go deeply within. Into your darkness. What is ready to grow, to become? Go deeply within. Surround yourself with this fertile darkness: *surrender—feel—explore—be.*

Breathe deeply in and out. Feel a gentle pull back from the depths of Mother Earth, from the depths of the void through the portal of your womb. You are back in your womb space now. Remember, this world is just a dream, and you are its dreamer. We are dreaming in the darkness, and you have the ability to dream your world into being. Breathe deeply into your womb. Now I would like to invite you to gather all the energy, all the wisdom from your womb and on the in-breath move it up into your heart space. On the out-breath move it back to your womb. Move this beautiful energy to your heart so you can feel your truth. Now on the in-breath, let's move this energy to the top of our head. On the out-breath move it back into your womb. Move this beautiful energy to the top of your head, so you can know your truth. Now on the in-breath, move this energy to the top of your head and on the out-breath move it down all over your body. Surround yourself with this energy like in a cocoon. Allow its medicine to penetrate you, and let it go. Let it flow where it wishes so. If into your body, let it be. If into Mother Earth, allow it to be so. If it spreads and flows into the world or disappears, just let it go. Gently, easily, and with trust. Breathe normally. Slowly bring yourself back. Introduce gentle movement into your fingers and toes. Stretch your arms and legs. Gently move and stretch your neck. And when you are ready, but only when you are ready, open your eyes. You are fully present, safe and at peace.

Questions to journal with

– How do I feel about the void?
– What does the void mean to me?
– What am I ready to let go of? What does no longer serve me?
– What is my gift growing in the darkness right now?
– Am I ready to let it grow?
– What is my medicine at this moment?

Goddess of the void—dancing with Hekate

Hekate is a liminal deity. She inhabits the places in between. She is one of the Dark Goddesses, Dark Feminine. The Dark Goddess has existed since storytelling began. The goddess of the underworld, goddess of death, ruling over everything we fear. But she is also the She Who Lights the Way—a hope carrying torches and lighting our way through the darkness. She likes nothing better than to break us apart, only to remake us anew. The Dark Goddess and the lessons she teaches are vital to our lives. She teaches us that there is death within life and that we are constantly changing and evolving. She is also the keeper of the dead and teaches us how to pierce the veil and see into the future. How to commune with our ancestors and how to become an ancestor when the time comes. Hekate was a Thracian moon goddess and was absorbed by the Greeks as a Titan. As we know from mythology Zeus—the Olympian God, fights and destroys the Titans, but not Hekate. She is too powerful for that. Originally, she is much more ancient and hence her power and strong will. She has the power of magic and sorcery. She is the goddess of the storms, wisdom, crossroads, borders, doorways, magic, the night, the warm abyss of the womb, witches, women, the void, the threshold between the worlds of the dead and the living—she is a truly primordial goddess with many aspects. She also is one of many names. *Nyctipolus* (night-wander), *Chthonia* (of the underworld), *Dadouchos* (torch-bearer), *Atalus* (tender, delicate) as well as flesh-eater, standing at the gate, protectress of children, and Triformis. She is often depicted in triple form and as such she is ruling over a wide range of influence in our lives and over our entire menstrual cycle. It was Hekate who assisted Demeter in her search for her daughter Kore, guiding her through the night with her flaming torches. It was also Hekate who became Persephone's guide and her companion while she dwelt in Hades. In her more vengeful aspects, she could unleash the hordes of demons and evil spirits on people and cities, but she could also deter harmful spirits from households and towns. Her sacred animals are dogs, horses, owls, and serpents. She is feared by many and still worshipped by many more.

As a liminal deity, Hekate is waiting for you at the threshold. She is there when you find yourself in between. She stands by you in the void, in the darkest night. She whispers to you in your dreams, in the hooting of an owl, in the barking of the dog at night. Her companionship is not easy. She will choose the most difficult road, the most inner route, but if you follow her you will find your inner strength and courage and you will tame the night and the fears and conditionings that night brings with itself. She will talk to you through your dreams, so look deeply into your night visions—the good ones and the ones of the scary kind. She is standing at the crossroads bearing the keys to the mysteries. She will inspire you and bestow her blessings. She will help you through transitions, she will protect you and guide you. As the Queen of Witches, she beckons you to trust in Nature, in the natural order of things and in your body. So, find your inner-witch, inner Wise Woman, and dive deeply into the void to hear her call.

Next time when you find yourself in the void find a quiet place at home or in nature, still your mind and body and go deeply within. Stillness and spaciousness are the key words for working with the void. When you find stillness without and within, you will be able to make space for the void and its message. Ground yourself by walking barefoot on the ground, or by simply sitting on the ground (or the floor in your house) and imagine roots growing from your legs into Mother Earth, anchoring you within her. When you feel grounded, drop down into your womb and just be. Without expectations, without any agendas, just be with yourself. Witness the void, the feelings it brings up to the surface, your emotions. Don't judge. Just witness. With kindness, compassion, and love for yourself. If tears come, let them. If any noises want to come through, allow them to come through your body. Be the channel, be the outlet for those emotions, words, feelings. And if you get unsure or scared, breathe deeply, and imagine Hekate standing there beside you with flaming torches in her hand. Allow the warmth and the light of the flame to penetrate the void, to scare the demons away. She is their mistress; they will listen to her command. Trust. Be. Allow yourself this space. The void doesn't like to be conquered, the void likes to be experienced. The more you fight against it, the harder its lessons will be. But if you soften and find stillness, you will discover the void as possibility, as the expanse. And in your own vulnerability, you will find an immense strength.

Void meditation with Hekate

Sit comfortably. Close your eyes and place one hand on your heart and one on your womb. Breathe deeply in and out. Feel your breath becoming longer and deeper, and as it happens so, allow your body to become more and more relaxed. Feel blissful heaviness spreading all over your body. Breathe deeply in and out. Take your time. When you feel relaxed step into your heart space. How would you like to do it? Would you like to float there gently with your in-breath? Or maybe just feeling the warmth of your hand on your chest will allow you to simply be transported there, within yourself? Just allow yourself gently to become present in your heart space. Breathe into your heart space. In and out. Bring life-giving breath into your heart space. Bring there your attention, your warmth and love. You don't have to do anything else. Just breathe there for a moment and be. Now, on the out-breath drop down into your womb space. Bring life-giving breath into your womb space. Bring there your attention, your warmth and love. You don't have to do anything else. Just breathe into your womb space and allow yourself to just be. Connect to your inner-most places. Connected to your true self. Breathe deeply in and out. And as you are breathing, invite your body into stillness. Notice how your body reacts to stillness. Does it feel uncomfortable or annoyed, does it want to move now more than ever, or does it settle into it with curiosity and gratitude? Whatever your body is feeling, send a message to your body that it is okay to feel that way. Give yourself and your body permission to feel that way. Breathe deeply, and when your body welcomes the quiet, allow yourself to drop fully into that divine stillness. Is your stillness surrounded by darkness or filled with light? There is no right or wrong way to feel this, there is only your body and your experience. Let go of all expectations. Let go of all the things you have going on in the outside world. Let go of your thoughts, feelings, wants, and needs. There is only stillness, emptiness, darkness, or light. There is only this sacred space. Pull all your precious energy from the outside inwards, back into your centre. Back into your heart. Back into your womb. You are the sacred space. Spend some time with this sacred you. With your Divine Feminine energy. And at any time if you start to feel lost or scared, feel, will or imagine Hekate's torches lighting your way back into your body, into your sacred space.

Now in your imagination see the candle flame flickering in the distance. Lighting your darkness or giving you a point of concentration through the light. Follow that flame, follow that light. You can see it growing bigger and bigger. This is Hekate's torch of courage. When you reach it take it into your hands and absorb it into your body. Feel the liquid fire dripping into your womb. Allow that to happen with trust. This is a fire of your courage, of your strength, that will stay dormant in your womb, and you will be able to activate it, to light it up and call its power whenever you are in need of courage. Whenever the void is too overwhelming and you'll find yourself lost in the dark, this flame will give you the strength and courage to go on or wait it through. Absorb the flame now. Feel it within your body. Feel it with trust. You are safe. Breathe deeply.

Now thank goddess Hekate, thank the flame, and thank your beautiful body. On the in-breath move your energy from your womb into your heart space. Once more fill your heart space with love and compassion. On the next out-breath step out of your heart space in the same way you stepped in there. Get back to feeling your entire body. Take a deep breath in and a deep breath out, maybe the deepest one you have done so far today. Introduce a little movement in your fingers and toes. Move your neck. Stretch your body. And when you are ready, but only when you are ready, open your eyes.

Welcome back. Now please take your journal and write down your experiences and thoughts.

CHAPTER 2

Menstrual wintering

The wintertime

Winter is the coldest season of the year. It is also the darkest one. The whole of nature is resting, sleeping off the business of summer and autumn. Animal larders are full, and their owners are retreating within their caves and burrows, huddling together for warmth and comfort. Some unlucky ones will go hungry. Some will die. Some are hibernating, suspended in a death-like sleep. There is not much activity in the outside world. The plants wither and die down, back into their seeds and bulbs, promising re-birth when the time comes. The trees stand naked, unembarrassed by their vulnerability and hope. All of Nature holds in her breath. There is silence and calmness in the air, but when the winter storm comes there can be destruction and tension. There are days when all seems bleak and dead. But there are also days when frost paints the most beautiful masterpieces on the leaves, cobwebs, and our windows. Days when the winter sun shines through the mists of our breaths. And warmly tucked under the blankets, the whole world is waiting, suspended in the promise of spring to come. Winter is necessary. Winter is a time of rest. It is a time of retreat. Winter is a time to go deeply down within yourself, to take stock, to get to know the real you and just simply be. It's a time to rest and to gather strength for the seasons to come. But we humans want to do things differently. As we get used to the electric lights, warm houses, and easy ways of transportation, we are treating winter as any other season. We are telling ourselves we can be super productive all year round and remain blind to the lessons from nature. Vulnerability, introspection, emotions, and our naked self are something that we tend to hide from the world and from ourselves. And I suppose winter is the time of hiding—from the frost, cold, and darkness, but we took it to a whole new level numbing ourselves and pushing forth. Is it really surprising then, that when the spring finally comes, we find ourselves absolutely exhausted? We find that we have no strength or the will to live. The depression statistics are starting to grow in springtime, and we just simply cannot find ourselves in the newly re-birthed world. Because as the world around us is so very much alive, we find ourselves descending into darkness and death, and this dissonance is sometimes too much to bear. But darkness and death are equally important, and we need to face them when the time is right. The postponing of the descent is what gets us in trouble. There are things in this life that we simply cannot escape. Even if we try to push it down into the fringes of our psyche and try to run from them with all our might, sooner or later the winter will catch up to us, and we'll find ourselves unprepared and absolutely overwhelmed. And then we will declare war on winter because that's what we do when we're frightened. And what chance do we have fighting with the seasons? What chance do we have in a fight with nature?

Women are wintering many times in a yearly cycle. There is a winter season that lasts from December to February, and the winter of our menstruation which we experience during each monthly cycle. There is also a 'winter' in the phases of the moon—it's when the moon is darkening and disappearing from our night sky. There is also the night—a beautiful time pregnant with possibility. They are all (the season, the menstruation, the moon, and the night) great tools that we are given to help us learn how to slow down, gather back the energy, and prepare ourselves for the re-birth of the spring, for re-entering the 'new day'. They are also all necessary for our mental and physical health. It breaks my heart when women are talked into stopping their menstrual cycle with a pill and promised non-stop productivity. It is not natural and not healthy, and sooner or later it will take a huge toll on their well-being. At the end of the day, should we try and stop winter from coming? Would we be really so much better off without it? I will leave the answer for you. So how does winter correspond with our menstrual cycle?

Wintering of menstruation

If you ever in your life menstruated, you would know this is the time when your energy is very low, you are tired, your womb is cramping its lining out of your body, and you just want to hide in the dark corner and hibernate until it passes. You need quiet and you often need to be still. Our modern lives are so hectic that many women do not allow themselves to bleed naturally. Their body is bleeding or craving a bleed, but a tampon or a pill will make them unaware of this fact, and they will carry on 'as normal', sometimes pushing even harder mentally and physically to earn their place in a male-dominated world.

Everyday life does not stop for menstruating women either. The demands of running a household and working for a living are over-whelming for all. This makes accepting the idea of menstruation as a winter break really difficult, especially if in their day-to-day life women are not allowed to slow down, not to mention to stop and listen. The modern woman is in need of a balance between her family life, work-load, and time to meet herself and her own needs. As the physical need of menstruation is to slow down, retreat, and go within, many women find this dissonance more than overwhelming. In a perfect world, we would have enough time to stop and look after ourselves. We would have our families on hand to help with kids and chores. But I'm not delusional, and we are not living in a perfect world. Does it mean we are all doomed? On the contrary. The change lies in our own hands. The change in how our society perceives women and the menstrual cycle. We *are* that change, and we *are* our attitudes and beliefs towards those subjects. If I would ask you now to close your eyes, breathe deeply and answer the question—how do you feel about your menstruation—what would you say? I love my bleed time. I love this powerful time given to me each month. Do you? Please let me explain why our men-struation is so amazing. Let's start with the blood itself. For centuries now menstrual blood was considered dirty, unclean, disgusting, and filled with shame. To this day in some cultures menstruating women are perceived as so unclean and polluting that they are forbidden to touch food and men. Menstrual blood is a taboo. But please stop for a moment and think about it. Your menstrual blood is composed of blood, vaginal fluid, and fluid and cells of the late secretory phase of the uterine endometrial lining, which is shed during your bleed. It is filled with stem cells (multipotent stem cells that are useful in tissue engineering and regeneration).

Your menstrual blood is filled with the possibility of life. Of life that hasn't come to be in a human form, but life, nevertheless. Your blood is filled with cells that create and maintain life. When you look at your menstruation like that can you still think of it as dirty and unclean? Blood used to be considered sacred. It was offered as an offering to gods and nature. Sometimes only blood could tame the raging deity. Your menstrual blood is the most sacred secretion your body produces. In some instances, the best blood offering was considered the blood of a virgin. However, there is research that suggests that the blood wasn't taken by taking the life of the virgin. It was taken from her menstrual blood. Menstrual blood was used in the manufacture of love charms and potions. It was used to ward off evil and protect livestock. It was considered powerful and surrounded by fear, myth, and legend. And so was a menstruating woman. In tribal times, menstruating women would gather in Red Tents or Menstruation Huts. They are present in some places of today's world as well, but their meaning has changed and degraded. Only by being marked as unclean, polluting, and shameful women are confined into the menstrual huts in Pakistan, India, Africa, and Nepal, to name just a few. They are not allowed to touch food, clothing, children, or men as they may pollute them in physical and metaphysical ways. They are rejected from and by society for the time of their bleed. But in the tribal times of the past, women would gather in the menstrual huts to bleed together in peace and calmness. They would spend time together, tending to their own needs of retreat, rest, and looking within. They would dream and connect with their oracular nature and see the future of their tribe through the prism of their blood. They would be taken out of their ordinary chores not because the bleeding would make them unclean, but to give them the time to rest and to mark the time of sacred ceremony. Because when we bleed, we are in ceremony. The chieftains would come to ask for advice. And bleeding woman wouldn't be touched by a man not because she could pollute him, but because she was considered sacred. She became the goddess and divinity is not touched by human hands. But his-story changed the meaning of the huts and added a few additional wounds to the feminine.

So next time when you are in ceremony, please ask your partner: do you know how much energy it takes for me to bleed? He won't know. But not because he doesn't care. He just simply has never been told before. His mother, sisters, and aunts kept menstruation a taboo, and they kept going even if they had to bite their fingers and grate their teeth. So, you tell him. Explain to him what it means to be a menstruating woman. How much effort it takes for your body, mind, and psyche. Ask him to help you. Ask him to take the kids to the park, cook dinner, massage your feet, or just let you be alone, in the darkness, feeling the flow, reconnecting with your inner-wisdom. Make this time sacred for both of you. Why not? Introduce new rituals. He loves you; he'll understand. I'm sure he would love to be able to help, to be included, to be invited into understanding this sacred concept he was excluded from for so many centuries. Your Divine Feminine needs his Divine Masculine and vice versa. And if you are in a relationship with a woman, talk to her all the same. Tell her how you are feeling, what would you like her to offer you for this sacred time, and what you are ready to offer to her. Communication is the key, learning together, getting to know each other, and understanding where we are and what is happening. Wouldn't you help the person you love? Then why do you think your partner wouldn't understand or wouldn't try to help as well? And be mindful that this shift won't happen overnight. It may take one cycle to change, it may take a hundred. But change is needed, and you are the change this world needs. But don't try to change all at once, it's never that easy.

Alexandra Pope and Sjanie Hugo Wurlitzer in their book *Wild Power* give the wonderful idea of a 1% change. This is a manageable amount for you and those around you. And when this 1% change becomes a norm introduce another 1%, and then another. And in that way before you know it your whole family will be on the same page, and you will be able to retreat into your inner winter in peace and with gratitude. And you can teach that to your children, daughters as well as sons, so the next generation knows. So, for the next generation it is not a taboo anymore. So, from the youngest age, they will learn how to talk about menstruation and through that how to talk and express their emotions and fears, even the most hidden ones.

Menstruation is our special time to connect to our deepest inner-wisdom. It is an oracle time, as we are channelling information from the spirit—as within so without, as above so below—and we are the chalice of that knowledge. If you are struggling with deciding about something, bleed on it. The answers will come with your flow. Menstruation is the time to dream. In dreamtime, we are the walkers between the worlds, between the times. We can connect to our ancestors and their wisdom. We can think and prepare for the new cycle. What is needed? What am I struggling with? What do I need to release? What do I crave for? This is the time of our intuition, of deeper knowledge. Therefore, journaling is so important. In this way you can receive from yourself, you can channel from the spirit, from the universe, from your ancestors. During our moon-time, the lower levels of oestrogen, progesterone, and basal body temperature make us feel heavy, gentle, vulnerable, and tearful. With the flow we become open to all, therefore we often feel the need to retreat, to cave in. And in the silence of our cave, we can hear all the messages better, louder. We can feel connected to something more. We can cleanse ourselves not only physically, but also energetically, spiritually, and emotionally. Through gentle pain we are shedding the past, again on all levels. Through contraction of our womb, we can release. Through breath, we can be born anew.

In winter everything becomes accessible and visible—there is no overgrowth to blind our vision. By inner seeing and listening we can allow ourselves to connect with our primal wisdom, with the goddess within. And so open we can interpret all the whispers from our guides, ancestors, universe, gods. We can allow the old to die together with our old cycle, and we can open ourselves to the birth of the new. We can grow and develop. We can truly become. And then we can welcome the spring filled with hope and energy. Because if we approach the spring without rest our energy levels won't be able to replenish. And then, how can you survive the entire next cycle? How will you be able to seek pleasure, to enjoy your life, family, work, and hobbies? Winter introduces mindfulness, the presence in the body, in your body. So be present; embody yourself. Embody your entire being. Through your menstruation, you are rising from the void. You are rising through the force and power that lies behind creation: pure feminine power. Going through the void supports the re-birth process, and supports the transformation. It connects us to the shadow, to the deepest grief and pain. It will enable us to surrender to feminine power, to accept it, to embrace it, to embody it. It can reveal deep wounding but also heal those wounds. This is the most potent, mysterious, and marvellous time there is. It is the time of open gates. When the flow pushes through our *Yonis* and the blood gains momentum, we are transported into the future but also into the past.

If you are struggling during your menstruation and have been checked for any underlying medical conditions, (although one doesn't cancel the other) and you've got a clean bill of health from your doctor, it may mean that travelling through the gate of the past can help you to resolve your struggle. The most common complaint of menstruation is pain. If you check with yourself and you've already changed your attitude towards your moon-time, you started to love and appreciate it, you are resting and flowing, meditating, dreaming, eating right, and practising your oracular gifts and the pain is still there, there may be another reason you would like to examine. Pain usually comes from inflammation. If there is no physical inflammation, there may be an emotional one. Menstruation takes us to the time of our birth. Like I've mentioned before, it is a time of death and re-birth that happens month after month. And if the re-birth of menstruation is hard to live through, we may want to look to the time when we entered this world ourselves for the first time in this life.

If your mum is still on this side of the veil, talk to her. Ask her about her birthing experience. What type of birth was it? The way we enter this world is crucial for us. So, ask her, was my birth on time or late, natural or assisted in any way? Were any painkillers or other medicines involved? How was her pregnancy with you? Where you a wanted pregnancy? What was she thinking about and what was she doing while pregnant? These conversations demand openness and courage. Please approach them with an open heart and compassion. Don't judge your mother. She was living her own life in the way she thought best. She was trying, exactly as you are trying now, her hardest. There is a lot of healing held within those conversations. But they may also open many wounds, so please be sure that both of you get help if you feel that appropriate. Talking therapy can move a lot of issues and open a free flow. But coming back to your birth—did you have an opportunity of skin-to-skin contact right after your birth? All those things are immensely important for processing and re-birthing. Think about it, how can you re-birth fully if the weight of the previous birth is pulling you down? One birth at a time, like peeling away the layers of an onion. Your menstruation is taking you back right into your own birth. Write down the birth experience of your daughter. Write it now when the memory is fresh. What happened, how long, what were you feeling, thinking? Were you scared? How did she come through? It will all influence her future *menses*. Write it down, as when your daughter will be looking for her answers, you may be already on the other side of the veil, without the possibility of sharing her truth with her. If you leave a written record, you will be able to remember everything yourself, but you will also make sure that if you pass on before her search begins, she will still be able to process it, to work through it, to let go, to heal.

Processing my own birth helped me immensely in taming the pain of adenomyosis. At the very beginning of my adventure with this condition, I felt lonely and petrified. The pain was debilitating. I would lose days because I was stuck in bed crying, fainting, not knowing what was going on and what to do. To be perfectly honest with you, there were times that I thought I was dying. Processing everything that has happened during my own birth helped me to tame the pain and fear, and allowed me to understand what, how, and why I felt the way I felt when the flair-ups happened. It helped me to become fully born so now I can travel through my mini-deaths and re-births with more consciousness, love, and compassion. It didn't heal the adenomyosis, but that was never the objective. Tracking and understanding my cycle helped me to learn how to live with this condition and how to make this time more bearable and sacred.

Dark feminine

Two wonderful books *Reclaim your Dark Goddess* by Flavia Kate Peters, and a cult work by Clarissa Pinkola Estes *Women Who Run with the Wolves* bring us closer to the idea of the Dark Goddess. Flavia Kate Peters writes:

> the Dark Goddess has existed since storytelling began. She is the goddess of the great void; she is she without the name and yet is every name … It is she who presides over the long, bleak winter months, and it is she who calls through the harshness of disappointment, sorrow, envy, anger, and other lower emotions.

But Peters is also showing that the Dark Goddess is more than coldness and death. She is a wise grandmother; she is the guide through hardships and life's transitions. And as death, decay, and destruction are a natural part of life, the Dark Goddess takes away the old, all that is no longer necessary, and makes way for something totally new. So, what is Dark Feminine? When I was meditating on this question, my womb sent me this beautiful message—'Darkness as bright as the Light and Light as dark as the Darkness. We are one'. Dark Feminine is an integral part of our life and is as important as the Light or bright part. Our world is driven by duality. Life and death, destroyer and liberator, growth and decay. Our journey begins in the dark—in the darkness of the womb of our mother, and in the darkness of the womb of the Cosmic Mother. From the darkness of the moon, a new cycle appears and from the darkness of menstruation a new menstrual cycle begins.

Dark Feminine is a very potent energy. Often it is the voice of your suppressed self. Dark Feminine is a mirror that reminds us of places where we have disengaged with our own selves. It becomes so much easier for us to see when we connect to our bodies, to our wombs. We live in a world of polarity. We need darkness to appreciate and love light and vice versa. Dark here does not equal bad or evil. Not at all. Our society and hundreds of years of conditioning made us to believe so. But dark equals mystery, your mystery. The darkness holds this mystery. The darkness of the womb creates life. *Dark Feminine is.* Often, when we feel and meet darkness, we automatically go into the resolution mode—I'm feeling this way, so how can I fix it? But because *Dark Feminine is*, you don't correct her, you are spending time with her. You don't do—you are. You become. You look into the mirror she is holding in front of you, and you see, truly, deeply. And it's scary, and it's hard. But this is the only way to be re-born. The process of re-birth is tough, frightening, and sometimes painful, but it always requires space-holding.

You hold that space for yourself, and you may ask others to hold it for you. Your cycle enables your physical, mental, and emotional presence as well. You must trust that you are never given the burden of something that you cannot carry, that is not meant for you. And as women we know—it doesn't happen just once; it is the journey of the spiral. Everything happens in cycles, but we are not running in circles like headless chickens. Every time we travel around the bend of the spiral and come into the time of re-birth, we are a different person—the circumstances are different, and so is the re-birth. We are letting the different old die and a different new be born. And here lies the magic of cycle tracking and cycle awareness. Knowledge is power; power conquers fear, so we don't have to be afraid anymore. Now we have tools to look the darkness and the Dark Feminine straight in the eye and say: *I know you. I recognise you. I welcome you. I love you. I see you. I am.*

CHAPTER 3

Dancing with goddesses: the Dark Feminine

Lilith

We all know the story of Eve—the first woman fashioned from Adam's rib. Created for man to serve and bear children. But how many of us know Lilith's story? Not so many, as our patriarchal tradition decided to forsake this rebel. Although she may be forgotten by Christianity, Judaism knows her name even though she is not spoken of that often. But Lilith was the true first woman—wife to Adam, created from the same matter he was. Created in equality with the man and given the power of choice, a voice, and independence, and Lilith made her choice. The story has it that she had had enough of lying underneath Adam during sexual intercourse, and when asked to change he refused, she decided to leave and start life on her own. When she left the Garden of Eden, devastated and miserable, Adam bent God's ear for so long until the Almighty sent three of his angels to bring her back. Legend has it she refused the angels, God, and Adam. She had had enough. During her journey out of Eden, she met Samael, the Fallen Angel, and started a new relationship with her new lover.

How does this patriarchal story end? Adam got a new wife, created from his rib, so she wouldn't have any rebellious ideas. Lilith, on the other hand, got cursed, the ability to bear children was taken away from her, and she became not only a demon herself, but also the mother of all demons—feared, cursed, and forgotten. Sadly, the world is populated with subdued and invisible women, with sexually curious Eves from the Garden. Even though we would think that after so many sexual revolutions we could call ourselves free, capable, knowledgeable, embodied deeply, and comfortable with our bodies … but can we really? Female sexuality and female bodies are still a taboo not only in the world but also in our culture. Even though we call ourselves a developed nation, for many the mystery of *Yoni* is hard to face. Patriarchy gives us three options—Virgin, Mother, and Whore. In some countries, the options are only two—the Virgin Mother and the Whore. Yet what lies in between the two polar opposites is covered with a shred of mystery, fear, and darkness. This is where female sexuality lies. I call it the void of Lilith. Let me talk to you for a moment about this void.

I believe we tend to think that our freedom rests with the number of sexual partners we can have. That we freed ourselves to pick and choose and that is enough. But what if I tell you that the true freedom lies in the deep knowledge of your own body, in living in accordance with your cycles, in living with pleasure and with expansion? If you have no knowledge about all the wonders I've mentioned above, can you really call yourself free? Remember that knowledge is power. Patriarchy figured that out a long time ago and started to burn all women who knew. And we became frightened of this knowledge—knowledge of the Burning Woman. But the need for it is ablaze in our hearts and in our bodies. It is time to answer this call. It is time to come back to basics—to come back to the real you. Sexual energy is the energy that gives us life—to all of us, men and women alike. It gives us spontaneity, creativity, and freedom of expression. It gives us pleasure in life, self-worth, and beauty. It gives us respect, tenderness, care, sensitivity, and compassion and expands our capacity. As you open to more pleasure you gain more confidence and general happiness. Your nervous system relaxes and moves you from survival to thriving. Your life and body begin to self-regulate. You tap into your being, into your body, you slow down, and you start to see the beauty that surrounds you. The practice of embodiment takes patience, takes time, and takes up space, but then suddenly you are starting to take up space as well. You give yourself permission; you release shame, stay open and curious; because you are such an interesting, beautiful, and amazing creation. And the path to this knowledge is paved not only with curiosity, but also with being kind and loving to yourself—as true love is cultivated from the foundation of self-love, self-discovery, and self-acceptance. You are perfect as you are! But who are you? Wouldn't you like to know? I would. Your body wisdom is a story of sensuality, of pleasure.

Sexuality is a key part of who we are, entangled in our everyday life. If we can feel the fire within, we can feel free in our life and we can conquer the world. And if we feel the fire within, we can claim our pleasure and we can start feeling that constant contraction doesn't really serve us. From there we can begin to move from contraction into expansion, and we can free ourselves to explore the true meaning of pleasure, of orgasm, of life. And then we become truly embodied within our lives, truly present; and we can start making truly embodied decisions. And then we know ourselves and our sacredness, and we understand the meaning of life. And the void of Lilith becomes the fullness of life itself. And from a demon stored in the darkest parts of your unconscious, you become yet again the fully fledged goddess—the goddess of your own realm, of your body, of your mind and of your sexuality; and then you can achieve it all and bring happiness to the entire world. Isn't it time we claimed our equality back? Isn't it time we re-kindled our inner fires? Isn't it time we came together as sisters to support each other and our growth? Isn't it time? I am ready to claim my rightful place! I am ready to embody my life! I am ready to meet Lilith! Are you? Will you join me? And meeting the sovereign and the power starts with blood.

Get to know your blood

Your blood is life, yet the taboo surrounding menstrual blood seems to be hard to break even for us women. Hopefully by reading everything I have written about blood so far, your attitude has begun to shift already. Wholeheartedly I would like to invite you to touch your menstrual blood. Consciously touch it. Take it on your fingers and rub it between them. Don't let anyone tell you what is appropriate or not—this is your body and your blood. Find Lilith within, find your inner rebel, and laugh at patriarchy right in the face. Reconnect with the innate knowledge and coding in this life-giving nectar. Touch your blood every time you're bleeding. Notice the difference in consistency, colour, and maybe smell. Take your blood on your finger and anoint your forehead. Something truly powerful happens when you do that.

Close your eyes and take time to feel the connection with the blood and beyond. Feel the wisdom of your ancestors transferred to you through your blood. If you would like to take it further, choose the symbol that means something to you and draw it with your blood on your face or body. Sleep like that and see what dreams this connection will bring. If you are using cloth period pads, collect the water after soaking them before washing them. Share this water with your plants at home and in the garden. Make it a conscious offering to Mother Earth, to your intentions, to your dreams. Get to know your blood and power hidden within. Find pleasure in connecting to it. Tame your fear and embarrassment, release the shame—remember, blood is life. Your menstrual blood is the most sacred secretion there is.

Hekate

Like I mentioned before, Hekate's faces accompany us throughout the entire cycle. She is known as *Triformis*, She of the Three Faces/Forms, but for me she has many more aspects. She is the Goddess of the Void, but she is also a strong personification of the Dark Feminine. And what is beautiful about her is that she is the light bringer. She carries torches that light the darkness for us. She can help us with the density and horror of the dark and unknown. She is also a midwife, and she can assist us in re-birthing ourselves over and over. As the goddess of witches, she is the deity of all women who are interested in mysteries and those who are choosing to remain blind and deaf. Hekate is a primordial force. She is the Mysterious Maiden, the Wise Crone, the Queen of the Underworld, the Guardian of the Unconscious, and the Midwife of Life. Hekate dwells in liminal spaces, in spaces in between. In the time between the old structure and the new one which hasn't yet been created. And through that, she has insight and power over both. She is waiting for us at the crossroads, holding her torches high, beautiful in her feminine power. For many centuries Hekate was demonised by not only religious conditioning, but also by patriarchy. We were led to believe that only youth is worthwhile, and that maturity and menopause are ugly and almost demonic in nature. Why? Because youth is easy to control, but maturity holds the power within. So, when you find yourself at the crossroads, call for Hekate's help, for her wisdom and strength. And when you feel yourself suspended in limbo, Hekate will help you to become consciously re-born.

I would like to invite you to this wonderful practice—the Conscious Birth ceremony—that I hope you will find helpful. Please do this ceremony during your moon-time, to properly acknowledge your arrival at this place in time, in your life, at whatever age you are. To reinforce with consciousness and validate your being and the beautiful gift of your life. But not the innocent life of a baby, but life as a powerful awakened woman that you are. Also, whenever you are going through a hard time in life, when you shed the old and await with anticipation or fear of the new—these are the times when you are walking the liminal space. When you recover from the illness, when you struggle with diagnosis, when you are facing a dreaded divorce, when you are becoming a mother, when you are crossing through the gate of the menopause, whenever you feel you are going through death and re-birth process, this is a ceremony for you. Call forth Hekate's power and let her lead you through the dark. Follow her light, and cross over.

Conscious birth ceremony

During this ceremony, we are going to be working with the Dark Feminine, with the symbolism of the womb cave, with burying the old to create a place for the new, with the earth, with directions and elements, with a Medicine Walk, with blood, and with Hekate. We are going to work with our creativity, our will, and our imagination. You can make Hekate as much or as little part of this ceremony as you wish. If you are working devotionally, create a prayer for the goddess asking her for guidance and protection. The intention of this ceremony is to acknowledge your conscious birth, the shedding of the old and with hope, love, and compassion creating a place for the new. Although the Medicine Walk can be done whenever you have an opportunity, or whenever you are willing, this ceremony is to be held at your moon-time, or if you don't bleed anymore during the dark moon or in the wintertime. Are you ready?

If you feel creative, I would like to invite you to create an effigy of yourself. Please use natural materials. You can cut your silhouette from a piece of paper, use clay, you can knit a little doll. If you don't feel creative at this moment in time, I would like to invite you to do a Medicine Walk. Find a beautiful place in nature, a place of significance to you, or a place that you feel drawn to or called by. Before you enter this place, stop for a moment, and bring yourself into a meditative state. This is a sacred walk; it should be done in a sacred way. Bring an offering with you that you can leave upon entry for the spirits of this place—it could be seeds, nuts, or cookies you have made. Your intention for this walk is to find an object that will represent you. Breathe deeply and when you feel ready begin your walk. Walk slowly, mindfully, breathing deeply and feeling the sacredness of this place and of your walk. At some point, you will feel drawn to an object that would like to represent you. It could be a stone, a stick, or a seed of a tree growing nearby. Find your object. Ask permission before picking it up, and when you pick it up leave in its place an offering. Try to find your object on the ground instead of cutting or pulling plants out. Before you leave your special place, thank the spirits of that place for the assistance you have received, stop for a moment, and bring yourself back from your meditative state into your everyday consciousness. Return home.

Take your effigy in your hands. Sit in a meditative state holding it near your heart space or at your womb space. Connect to your womb. From this place of being, please take your menstrual blood and put it on your effigy. If you don't bleed anymore, you can use your hair or saliva. Find a place in nature you would like to hold your ceremony. It could be in your garden, in the park, in the forest. If you have your special place in nature that would be perfect as well. You can even come back to the place you have found your effigy in. At your special place dig a little hole (big enough to house your representation). Breathe deeply. Look at your effigy and say: 'This is I … [put your name here], and I'm consciously giving the old me into the safekeeping of Mother Earth. In the cave of your womb, Great Mother, I will be re-born anew'. Place the effigy in the earth and bury it (preferably using your hands). When you have done it, stand up, face the East and say:

> I'm calling in the East and sacred element of Air. I'm taking in my conscious breath and I'm filling my body with life-giving air [take the conscious breath]. May Air bring me new beginnings and teaches me to fly. I accept my new breath.

Now face the South and say:

> 'I'm calling in the South and the sacred element of Fire. I'm consciously lighting the spark of the spirit within my body. I honour my passion, creativity, and love, and I'm opening myself to them'.

Now face the West and say:

> I'm calling in the West and sacred element of Water. I'm consciously feeling the sacred waters flowing through my body—my tears, my sweat, my blood pulsating in my veins, and my menstrual blood flowing through my *Yoni*. I'm honouring the flow, transformation and femininity within me and I'm opening myself to them.

Now face the North and say:

> I'm calling in the North and the sacred element of Earth. I'm consciously inhabiting my body, every part of it. I'm honouring my ancestors, my maternal and paternal lines, and I am grateful for all the gifts I have received. I am thanking them for my precious life.

Now look up and say:

> I'm calling in the Great Above—Grandfather Sun, Grandmother Moon, and Father Sky, I'm consciously allowing the song of life to sound through me, through my body and my soul'.

Now kneel, touch the earth, and say:

> I'm calling in Mother Earth, her gift, her medicine, her presence, and through the cave-womb of her body I'm consciously being born. Through the offering of my blood, I am connected to you, Dear Mother. I step firmly on the ground; I know myself and my path. I am grounded, I am safe, I am loved.

Stand up and put your hands on your heart.

> I'm calling in the Great Within—midway between Heaven and Earth, to witness my conscious birth. I'm calling Hekate to be my witness and I'm asking her to light the path ahead. I am born now. I am born. I am born.

Feel each word deeply within. Acknowledge the shift in energy. Acknowledge your feelings and emotions. Flow with them. When you feel ready give your thanks to directions and elements, to the darkness of the moon, to the spirit of your effigy and the life past, to your re-birth process, to your ancestors, to your family, to the night/or day of your ceremony. Thank the Gods if you are so inclined. You can stay a little longer contemplating the place of your birth, thinking of the new you and all the possibilities unfolding in front of you. And when you feel complete, slowly, and consciously make your way home.

Kali

Hindu Goddess Kali is the essence and the primal symbol of universal life. She consists in herself the sacred duality of being a destroyer and a liberator. She is the greatest manifestation of Shakti (primordial, cosmic energy) and the mother of all living beings. Kali's myth says that Goddess Durga was attacked by some demons. A ferocious battle took place. Goddess Durga was overtaken by such anger for the insult that her face became all dark and Kali appeared out of her forehead. Kali immediately defeated some of the demons, but one—Raktabija—seemed to be undefeatable because of his ability to reproduce himself from every drop of his blood that touched the ground. Innumerable demons appeared on the battlefield. Kali, filled with her power, sucked all his blood before it could reach the ground and ate all his clones and in this way defeated him once and for all. Kali was ecstatic. She began to dance the dance of the victorious. But she was filled with the demon blood and the blood began to affect her. She danced more and more wildly, without pause, without consideration. Her dance started to create thunder and lightning and began to cause great destruction. Worried gods went to Shiva, Kali's husband, to ask him to calm her down. He tried, but she couldn't hear him. She was in a trance, deep within herself. Her primordial energy was displayed in all her power and fury. In an act of desperation, Shiva threw himself under her feet. Kali trampled on her husband, and all seemed to be almost lost, but suddenly she realised what she was doing and who was lying underneath her feet. Only that could bring her out of this trance. Only that could stop the destruction.

When you meet Kali, you are faced with the dark. But in the depths of that darkness, you can find the truth of who you really are. Kali's energy destroys, but only all that she is supposed to destroy. She cannot destroy anything that is true to you. Only things in dissonance with you will perish. Through dancing with Kali, you will be faced with your disowned self. But by recognising it, she will release your heart from its bounds, and you will be filled with your primordial energy—the energy of creation. Although destruction may look messy and violent, this is also a process of creation. When you consider the processes that belong to Kali you will be able to understand the meaning behind them. Birth belongs to Kali—and although the process of birth is filled with blood, pain, threat of death, sometimes anger, fear, the unknown, and bodily messiness—at the end of that creative process, you will hold a beautiful baby in your hands.

This is a true Kali transformation, as during birth nature takes over, the primal force, and your ego must step down. Kali will show you what is indestructible within you. She will destroy the false ideas you hold about yourself and the world around you. She may break down the karmic cycle. But she also teaches us about the importance of masculinity. The beautiful masculine is presented through the men in our lives, but also through the important inner masculine within every woman. The masculine is a container to hold the feminine. She is allowing us to understand that feminine energy may be chaotic, and untamed, and that's okay. There is nothing wrong with that. And by embracing the masculine (and the inner masculine) we are able to direct that flow. Without this masculine container, the feminine may sometimes get out of control and may fall into chaos. These are difficult lessons to learn, yet they are so very important.

Questions to journal with

- What parts of myself I am denying?
- What is preventing me from living in my power?
- Am I ready to allow some things in my life to go, so I can find my truth?
- What things in my life I am ready to let go of, and what things I must let go of?
- What does wintering mean to me?
- What are my tools for good wintering?

Fire practice

You will need a candle and a quiet place, preferably in darkness.

Sit comfortably and close your eyes. Centre yourself. Bring your attention to your body, drop down to your womb. Call upon Goddess

Kali for support. Ask her to come and sit with you as you are burning in the flame of the candle all that needs to be destroyed within you. Can you see her face? Can you feel her presence close to you? Can you feel the presence of the Dark Feminine.

Open your eyes and light the candle. Look into the flame. Hold your body. Feel Kali's presence holding you. Soften your gaze, breathe gently, and watch the flame. Become one with the flame. Find your rhythm—breathing, watching, maybe moving with the flow of the flame. Trust that the fire will transform any dense energies in your body that are obstructing your freedom, your joy of life. You don't *do* the Dark Feminine—you *are the Dark Feminine*. So be now. Just be. Watch the flame and be present.

When you feel complete with just being and watching the flame, take a deep breath in and with this breath call for Kali's support, wisdom, and love. Breath out through your mouth and with the exhale surrender to the power of the Dark Feminine (whatever it means to you). Please repeat this three times. Blow out the candle.

All is working out for your highest good. The universe has your back.

Repeat this exercise whenever you'd like to work with Kali, whenever you feel the need to connect with the Dark Feminine, and to connect to the wisdom of your blood at moon-time.

Including the masculine

It is very important to awaken your inner masculine, but it is equally important to connect to the masculine already present in your life. Your husband, boyfriend, partner, and son, all can be a container to hold you when you struggle, when you need support. They don't know they can do it because nobody ever told them that. You may be the first woman in their life to open the gate to the mysteries and wonders of the menstrual cycle. Be that woman; be that teacher. Teach them how to help you, what are your needs, and what comforts you require. Talk to them about your cycle. About the changes your body is going through, about death and re-birth. Be the priestess of the mysteries. Tell them how much energy it takes you to bleed. Ask them to cook for you then, to bring the hot water bottle, blanket, or socks. Ask them to cuddle you when you are in pain or to leave you alone if that's what you need. The masculine has its own rhythm too. There may be times that your partner will need a hug or to be left alone—agree on the way you will communicate that to each other, so everything is clear. So, neither of you feel hurt if the other one asks for space. Communication is the key. Open yourself to give and to receive, to understand each other and your needs. To fulfil them to the best of your abilities. Be the partner that you need. Allow him to hold you, to be your anchor, but at the same time put clear boundaries in place. For both of your sakes. Arrange 'me' time, so he can pick the kids up, and look after the dog, and you will have space to meditate, do your practices, and meet with your women's circle.

Explore, be curious, and come back to this conversation over and over again. Learn from each other. Flow together. Remember, feminine needs masculine and vice versa. You have them both within you. We all do. It's time to connect and channel this energy for the good of us all.

PART 2

THE RISE OF THE MAIDEN

CHAPTER 4

The wisdom of transitions

Nature is in constant flow—constant movement. The change in the flow and the movement comes through transitions. A transition is a transformation. As humans, we all have different needs that lead us to transform and progress, to keep the movement going. We all have different emotions, we grow, develop, and progress in different ways. But we also have similar patterns. And those patterns are visible in the transitions within our menstrual cycle. Our menstrual cycle trains us in transitioning and this is a training that adds so much wisdom to our daily lives. There are four main transitions in our menstrual cycle. Four transitions generally, but individually we may experience more, so always approach this teaching with an open heart and curiosity. Track your cycle passionately. I first heard about transitions from Melanie Swan when I was going to her Womb Medicine Woman Training, and this knowledge has changed my life.

Transitions have a very important purpose. The first transition occurs when we are flowing through menstruation to pre-ovulation. This transition is preparing us to meet the outside world again. The second transition weaves pre-ovulation to ovulation and prepares us to work on a different dimension, with a different energy level. It places us fully within the world. The third transition between ovulation and pre-menstrual helps us to gather back all the energy that we have sent into the world. It calls for the time for reflection and analysis. The fourth transition—pre-menstrual to menstrual—helps us to detach ourselves from the outside world. It prepares us for the womb cave, for silence. It helps us to rejuvenate our energy and to communicate beyond the veil. Each transition prepares us for the next phase of our menstrual cycle. As our cycle is a great feedback loop, each transition and how we manage it informs our presence in the next phase of our cycle, and each cycle phase informs each transition.

The first transition happens when we emerge from our moon-time. In a 28-day cycle, it usually occurs around days 6–7. If you allow yourself to rest during your menstruation, you will feel the desire to emerge. Again, if you don't allow that rest, there will be no desire to emerge, and your cycle will begin as if running on empty. This transition is holding the energy of self-care. Look for answers in nature, into hibernating animals. They don't just jump out of their caves and burrows. They move slowly, experiencing the world at a slower pace. They are tasting the air, stretching, and feeling their bodies after a long time of sleep. Be a bear experiencing the spring after the winter. Be gentle with yourself and mindful. On the first day of your cycle, the energy is at its lowest. From this point, the energy is going to expand and grow, and you together with it. The pick of your energy will happen at ovulation, and after this highest point in the energetic life of your cycle, the energy and you together with it will start to contract and go down, inwards, into the lowest point again. Rise and fall, expansion and contraction, in constant dance and weave. Only by being receptive to the flows and ebbs of your energy and the phase you are in, will you be able to be receptive to the entire world.

The second transition proclaims your energy going out. This phase usually lasts from days 7–12, with transition at days 10–12. This is the time of the Maiden. You've received the green light to go out and explore, to put yourself out there. This is the time of spring, flowers are in blossom, and everything is filled with life. But remember that each flower blossoms in its own time and opens its petals slowly and carefully. This is the time when your creativity is coming through, and you think there is nothing you can't do. The most important thing you can do to help yourself is to remember to remain grounded. Keep your feet firmly on the ground when your soul soars.

The third transition welcomes the energy back. These cycle days are usually between days 12–21 with transition anywhere between days 16–21. This is the time of not only welcoming the energy back but also grounding it in your own body. This transition can be deeply healing, as we can utilise and absorb all that we have learnt from being out in the world. But, if not managed, we can become very argumentative, and annoyed. This is the window to the parts within us that need to be seen and acknowledged.

The last transition will help us enter the void. These cycle days are 22–28 with the transition on days 27–28 (if your cycle is longer or shorter, it would be the last day before your bleed—the 28-day cycle is not the perfect cycle—it's only an example I'm using here). This is the time of nesting, and preparing for the retreat. You gather yourself in before you plunge into your void and through the lowest point of your energetic cycle, you will allow the old to die preparing a place for something new. If you won't slow down in your pre-menstrual phase, through the feeling of anger, frustration and rage, you will be thrown into the deepest of the voids. But don't despair, there is healing there too.

As each transition informs us about the phase we have just gone through and gives us the window into the phase we're just approaching, they also give us an opportunity to re-adjust, to change and get our cycle back on track. You don't have to wait for a new cycle to make it better, you can do it here and now. Isn't that a real blessing? Our body asks us for a lot, but only ever for things that are important. So, acknowledge your transitions, find time to rest, slow down, give yourself space to dream, do things step by step, not all at once, pay attention, reflect, emerge, and then when the time is right go back within. Track your cycle with compassion and kindness. Watch. Observe. When is your transition time?

Questions to journal with

- What are you willing to let go of?
- What are you trying to hold on to?
- How can you make it easier?
- What tools do I already have within?

Potions for transitions

Essential oils and herbs are a wonderful aid in times of transition. A calm nervous system is the foundation of any inner work. I'd like to invite you to try making some blends yourself. They will also make lovely gifts.

Essential oils for diffusers

Midnight stroll (for transition, when you feel down, when needing self-love and peace)

– 7 drops of Lavender
– 6 drops of Bergamot
– 6 drops of Frankincense
– 2 drops of Sandalwood

Put into a diffuser filled with water, breathe, and enjoy.
   Lethargy be gone (for the transition when you feel overly exhausted)

– 4 drops of Clary Sage
– 3 drops of Black Pepper
– 3 drops of Ginger

Put into a diffuser filled with water, breathe, and enjoy.
   Monkey mood (for transition with mood swings)

– 3 drops of Clary Sage
– 4 drops of Chamomile
– 5 drops of Lavender
– 3 drops of Sandalwood

Put into a diffuser filled with water, breathe, and enjoy.
   The flow (for transition when you find it difficult to stay positive)

– 3 drops of Basil
– 3 drops of Marjoram
– 4 drops of Ginger

Put into a diffuser filled with water, breathe, and enjoy.

The great empty (for the transition when you need your mind stimulated)

– 4 drops of Lemon
– 4 drops of Geranium
– 4 drops of Frankincense

Put into a diffuser filled with water, breathe, and enjoy.

The healing breath (for the transition when you need to release mental stress and calm the nerves)

– 3 drops of Lemon
– 5 drops of Lavender
– 2 drops of Ylang Ylang
– 4 drops of Frankincense
– 2 drops of Patchouli

Put into a diffuser filled with water, breathe, and enjoy.

Herbal infusions

Meadow of peace

Combine equal parts:

– Chamomile (*Matricaria recutita*)
– Lemon balm (*Melissa officinalis*)
– Lavender (*Lavendula officinalis*)

Mix all the herbs well. To prepare, put a large teaspoon of herbal mixture into a strainer, place it in your cup and pour hot water over your herbs. Make sure your strainer is large enough so your herbs can float and mix freely releasing all their goodness. Cover the cup, so the steam and all the essential oils stay in and let steep for ten minutes. Drink hot, inhaling the steam as you do so, as the steam has all the essential oils and will aid the relaxation process. You can drink this mixture as needed in stressful moments, 1–3 cups per day. This blend will aid general relaxation, relieve stress, and will promote a good night's sleep.

Please check with an herbalist or your doctor if you are pregnant or breastfeeding.

Into Morpheus's arms

- 1 teaspoon of Chamomile (*Matricaria recutita*)
- 1 teaspoon of Passiflora (*Passiflora incarnata*)
- ½ teaspoon of Skullcap (*Scutellaria leteriflora*)

This is my favourite blend for sleeplessness. One cup in the evening before bed brings me right into Morpheus's arms (hence the name). Chamomile eases muscle tension and is a very well-known sedative and relaxant. Passionflower is also a mild sedative and is very helpful in combating nervousness, restlessness, and sleeplessness and both of them are irreplaceable in helping with nervous gastrointestinal disorders—especially in children. Skullcap is gentle and nourishing to the nervous system, it helps to relieve occasional tension and stress, and is priceless for helping to calm worrying thoughts. It helps to relieve anxiety and insomnia.

To prepare put herbs into a strainer, place in your cup and pour hot water. Make sure your strainer is large enough so your herbs can float and mix freely releasing all their goodness. Cover the top, so the steam and all the essential oils stay in your cup and let steep for ten minutes. Drink hot inhaling the steam as you do so, as the steam has all the essential oils and will aid the relaxation process. Drink one cup half an hour before bedtime.

DO NOT USE THIS BLEND IF YOU ARE ON ANTIDEPRESSANTS OR SEDATIVE MEDICATIONS! Please check with your herbalist or doctor if you are pregnant or breastfeeding.

Simple solution

- 1 teaspoon of Chamomile (*Matricaria recutita*)
- 1 teaspoon of Skullcap (*Scutellaria lateriflora*)
- ¼–½ teaspoon of Peppermint (*Mentha piperita*)

Skullcap is gentle and nourishing to the nervous system, it helps to relieve occasional tension and stress and is priceless in helping to calm worrying thoughts. It helps to relieve anxiety and insomnia. Chamomile eases muscle tension and is a very well-known sedative and relaxant. Peppermint will add more flavour to your tea.

To prepare put herbs into a strainer, place in your cup and pour hot water. Make sure your strainer is large enough so your herbs can float and mix freely releasing all their goodness. Cover the top, so the steam and all the essential oils stay in your cup and let steep for ten minutes. Drink hot inhaling the steam as you do so, as the steam has all the essential oils and will aid the relaxation process.

This tea can be used throughout the day during stressful situations or at night before bed to calm worried thoughts.

STOP TAKING SKULLCAP 2 WEEKS BEFORE SCHEDULED SURGERY. Do not take if pregnant or breastfeeding.

CHAPTER 5

Maiden unleashed

The springtime

As the year turns and the seasons flow, spring follows winter with warmer days, shorter nights, and with the noise of nature returning to life. Everything is awakened—animals, plants, even us humans. Everything ventures out, to see and discover what new is coming. Spring is the time of re-birth, re-entering the world after the period of rest and seclusion. On wobbly feet, new life is welcomed on earth and young eyes can see for the very first time. So are we, seeing the world renewed, rebuilt, almost like we've never seen it before. Our senses are shocked by the colours, smells, by the warmth of the sun on our bodies. We take off our coats and this act in itself is almost equal to a re-birthing experience. Shedding off the old and getting ourselves ready for the new. We venture out. We become curious, more adventurous, and more conscious not only of our inner world, but of the one outside as well. From time immemorial the egg was the symbol of spring. It is associated with hope, birth, and resurrection. The Cosmic Egg is present in the mythology of many cultures, and it always takes us back to the beginning of the universe. And in your springtime, your ovaries are working hard to mature the egg that will be released in your summer. They are creating your inner universe, your inner miracle, the inner beginning. Another symbol of spring is the child or the maiden holding flowers. Spring is the conception, the genesis. Spring is the fresh air and innocence. Spring holds the promise.

The Maiden

In your Maiden phase, you enter your inner spring. It is a time when you start bringing your subconscious to the light of the day. It is a time of release of all the ideas that were incubating in the cave of your Dark Feminine. The Maiden has a gift of regeneration, resurrection, and renewal. This is a time of new energy and of incredible enthusiasm towards oneself and all of life. After the flow of your bleed, you are able to embody yourself once more. Your body becomes important and through your menstrual blood it is renewed. It is stronger, more vital, more confident, and filled with energy. Everything is bright and new, even your sexual nature. Everything becomes more fun-loving, flirta- tious, and outgoing. You are stronger physically and mentally. You can create space for new projects, as you feel more independent and your belief in yourself and in success is much stronger now. You feel ready to meet people once more, to go out, to share, to explore. You embody the pleasures of life itself. Your Maiden time is when the ideas cooked in your womb during your bleed are formed in a more physical way and given structure. From here you can push them forth. You can give them new light and new possibilities. This is one of the most dynamic phases in your cycle. But this is also a phase in which you can lose yourself. You may push forward too hard and allow your inner masculinity to take over. Without the inner-balance you may struggle with being over- achieving, and too self-sufficient and through that you may find it too difficult to surrender and to soften. It may take its toll on your relation- ships with yourself and others. And you may forget that you are still in need of self-care and caring for loved ones.

The Maiden brings the first stages of intimacy and touch: discovery of your own body, mapping the curves of it; the purity of your body and mind; innocence, playfulness, joy, happiness, peace, and clarity; freshness and growth; ideas and needs.

The Maiden phase is also a time for your inner-child. Find her, support her, give her a voice, and through that allow her to become. Mother her in a way she hasn't been in the past or in a way she needs to be mothered now. What is your inner-child telling you? What is she asking you to do? Hold her in the way she needs to be held. Be patient. Give her time and attention. Working with your inner-child is especially important if you are struggling with your Maiden phase. If you cannot find that freshness, that joy of life, this phase may trigger emotions and experiences from the past. But remember, the Maiden is not an outside force. This energy is coming from within you. This is you. You from the past and you from the present. You are all the phases. Deep within, you hold all the archetypes. Open yourself and listen to the wisdom within. Your wisdom. If your inner-child needs mothering, connect to the mother archetype within. Embrace that little girl, acknowledge her. You have all the tools. If she needs another child to be playful with, connect to your inner-child from the present. Allow your past child and your present child to play together, to roam free, to discover, to explore. Embrace her in this way and see what a difference in your adult life it will make. All your phases know each other, like you really know yourself, even though you may not be aware of that. As an example allow me to let you in on my own experience. Today, although I'm writing about the Maiden, I'm doing this from the perspective of the Crone. This is the energy I am in today. But my Crone knows my Maiden. It is all me. It is all I. Breathe deeply, connect to your body, and answer this question. Where in your body does your Maiden live? Is it in your head, heart, hands, or womb? Look deeply. Where does she hide? My Maiden lives in my heart. This is very interesting as this is the place where my Crone lives as well. I think sometimes my Crone looks after my Maiden like a good grandmother.

The symbol of my Crone is the spider. The symbol of my Maiden is the butterfly. The butterfly is the symbol of transformation, it is the water, emotions, flow, femininity, sensuality. Spider is the earth—it's grounding, stability, growth, fertility, but also death and decay. Polar opposites, perfect union. Maiden comes out through the door in my head, although she lives in my heart. Crone comes directly from her heart cave. They both hold their wisdom. They are both filled with strength. They are both there when I need them. So, I can draw on the wisdom of my Crone when my Meiden needs it most. I can ask my inner-mother to come forth if that is what is needed. But it works both ways, sometimes when my Crone gets too lost in the darkness, my Maiden comes to the rescue, with shining torches, with freshness and laughter. Remember, all that wisdom is already within you. We are just creating easier access to it.

Maiden energy is open to the Beauty Way. She brings beauty to every situation you are in. When things get ugly, she brings integrity and peace to the situation. She creates beauty in your life and recognises beauty in yourself and others. She takes time to stop and smell the flowers, to breathe, to run and to dance. She lifts her head and sees the stars. She sees the world with a fresh gaze. Maiden is that part of you who still believes in magic. Who speaks to the trees, rivers, ocean, and spirits. She can see them all as well and her innocence hasn't been tainted yet. Maiden knows the way to joy and happiness. She offers you the return of the second innocence, but one born of wisdom not of naivety. She can help you to acquire a beginner's mind so that you can see all as if for the first time. She is calling you to remain open, to learn and discover.

If you find this phase very difficult, go back in the timeline of your life to your childhood and check what happened to you then. Were you subjected to sexual assault, violence, trauma? Did you have an accident? Did you lose a loved one? Or maybe your favourite pet? Did you feel heard and acknowledged during your childhood and teenagerhood? The Maiden is a mirror of that time in your life-cycle. She may be showing you things that haven't been processed yet. Maybe you are ready to process them now. Please find the right recourses, counselling, and therapy, and see what your Maiden is showing you. Give her back her voice. Hear what she is telling you. Maybe you will be the first person who will allow her to truly express her needs and pain. Maybe you will be the first person who will see that pain and will do something about it. Believe me, the healing that will arise from there is deeper than you can imagine.

Another thing that can impact how you are feeling during your Maiden phase is what happened to you during your *Menarche*. *Menarche* is the time of your first blood, the moment you menstruate for the very first time. In the olden days, this was a very important rite of passage in a woman's life and was celebrated by the whole community. Today, it's forgotten, unimportant, and shrouded in taboo. In our culture rituals have lost their meaning. But humans are ritualistic. We have the daily rituals we follow faithfully, the annual ones we observe, for example, your birthday. We just took the sacred out of them. We have religious days and celebrations. Each Christmas or Easter, each New Year's Eve, we follow certain practices and couldn't imagine our lives without them. Yet, something as important as a change in status—from a child to a woman, is unmarked and unnoticed. But the life of that little girl at that moment changes dramatically.

As we are living in a society that doesn't talk about periods, this little girl approaches that change not only unprepared, but also very often without adequate support. And that opens the gates of fear, shame, inadequacy, disgust towards one's body, and feelings of loneliness and of being lesser than those who don't bleed. And for the rest of her life, that girl will bleed alone. It's the right time to break that process. To claim the proud feeling of becoming a woman, a creatrix of life, an adult. Let's create a celebration for this transition into womanhood. Let's get together, sing, dance, and tell stories of the blood. But not the scary stories; you must remember that a healthy menstrual cycle is not something to dread. And a healthy approach to it can open the gate to a wonderful adventure in meeting and getting to know the real you. So many women in my generation, in generations of my mother and grandmothers didn't have an opportunity of celebrating this moment. Luckily, we can still through ritual and ceremony go back in time and repair it. We can celebrate our womanhood, and our sisterhood together, and create new rituals for our daughters to pass onto them as their new inheritance. Because how can we fully embody ourselves if we haven't welcomed all the parts? If we haven't truly arrived in our own life. If we haven't fully acknowledged and processed what is happening to us and our bodies. How can we accept our cyclicity if we haven't welcomed it in the first place?

I've created this *Menarche* Ceremony for the women in my *Yoni* Wise groups. The healing that this ceremony weaved into their lives is so immense that I have decided to share it with you in this book. I know from my own experience the importance of a *Menarche* Ceremony regardless of age. When I accepted that part of me and welcomed her into my life, something shifted deep within me. I felt more acceptance and peace towards myself and my body. By then I already loved my blood, but this ceremony deepened this love in a way I didn't think possible. I felt completed, fully arrived in my body, it felt as if everything got back to its proper place. It felt like a soul retrieval. In a way, I believe this ceremony is a soul retrieval. As I welcomed back this frightened little girl, she returned with an incredible amount of strength and purpose. And she completed me as an adult woman. And she showed me the innocence and the sacredness of this process. And this is what I would like to share with you now.

To create your *Menarche* Ceremony you will need intention, will and imagination. You will also need a group, or at least one other woman. If you could find three other women that would be perfect. You could divide the ceremony into two. The two of you would hold it for the other two, and then you would swap. You will need to find a space to hold your ceremony. It could be outside in nature, in your living room or you could rent a place if you feel it appropriate. You would need flowers, candles, and beautiful objects to make it a special and sacred space. You could invite other women to witness your ceremony—your daughters, sisters, aunts, friends. You could invite your mother or a grandmother if that is what you wish. You could prepare lovely food to share with everyone afterwards. For my ceremony, I created an altar. I put on it one red candle and one white, incense, smudging sticks, feathers, water, earth or salt, flowers, and something from nature that symbolises the season we are in at the time of our ceremony.

For each participant, I ask them to prepare a red candle, a letter that they deliver to me before the ceremony and a token. The token will be a reminder of this ceremony. It will be something you can wear or use every time you are bleeding—so it can remind you of the time you were in the sacred space with other women. When you were held in safety and highest regard. It could be a piece of jewellery (neckless, ring, bracelet), a stone, a shawl, or anything you can think of and then use as a reminder. I also ask all my participants to write a letter to themselves. In this letter I ask them to put everything that this little girl who has just started bleeding would like/need to hear, and everything they as adults would like to tell her. I receive those letters before the ceremony, and I learn how to read them beautifully for them. I have found that writing a letter to your litter girl is really healing and transforming, but having those words read by someone else during the ceremony is even more powerful. The last thing you will need is the flower crown. Remember you are returning to your Maiden phase, so make her as beautiful as you dare.

One last thing—find or write a poem that would be appropriate for this occasion. Poetry has a way of penetrating our hearts and souls and getting right there to the depths of our being. So go for it, allow your Maiden to take you for an adventure. Don't feel embarrassed, just write, whatever she is whispering in your ear. Now you are ready for the ceremony. Pick a date and invite your women tribe.

In this ceremony, you are going to go back in time. I am using the sound of the drum to take us there. You are going to walk back to the time of your first bleed. The ceremony will happen there. If you have guests witnessing, they won't go back. They will stay in place holding the sacred space for you. The main part of the ceremony will happen in the past—the welcoming, the acknowledging, the letter reading. Then you will travel back to now. To today, here, and now of your normal life, to the moment in which you have begun your ceremony. And when you return you can be welcomed by the witnessing women, and you can share the feast and experiences. Have a beautiful journey.

Menarche *Ceremony*

Prepare the space and your altar. Light the candles. Ask the participants to put flower crowns and their tokens on the altar.

Welcome everyone and smudge them in. (You can use sage, lavender, incense, and a rattle to rattle everyone in). Create a sacred space. (All my ceremonies are shamanic in nature, so I always call in directions and elements, my guides and allies, ancestors and lineage, the spirits of nature, and of course the spirit of the Cosmic Womb).

Connect to your womb and lead everyone to connect to theirs.

Stand in the circle. (If you have guests, create an inner circle for participants of the ceremony and an outer circle for the guests)

Say out loud:

Let us take a few breaths together. In through your nose, out through your mouth.
Let's take our first breath with the Earth.
Let's take a second breath with the Sky.
Let's take a third breath with the Sea.
Let's take a fourth breath with the Fire within and without.
Let's take a fifth breath with our ancestors.
Let's take a sixth breath with this circle and all the women present here today.
Close your eyes and feel the presence of All.

Now holding your drum or a rattle begin to walk anticlockwise. Drum or rattle a beat for your journey. We are going back in time now. You are going back to the time of your first bleed. It will be different for each of us. As you walk feel your years are falling down like the leaves. Breathe deeply and allow them to fall. And with each falling year you become younger and younger. Until you reach the time of your first bleed. Using your intention, will and imagination arrive at the time of your first bleed.

When you feel you have reached the right time, stop walking. (Remember, only the inner circle is walking, the guests are witnessing).

We have gathered here today to celebrate our Menarche Ceremony. To celebrate us—women, maidens, daughters, mothers. To celebrate us, our cyclicity, femininity, sexuality, our bodies, and our wisdom. Welcome to the Circle of Women.

Approach each participant separately:

- Put a bit of earth on their feet and say—'May the earth always support you'.
- Circle her head with the feather and say—'May you grow wings to help you soar'.
- Put water on her hands and say—'May this water bring you health and life'.
- Light their candle with the red candle from the altar and say—'May this light always illuminate the dark for you'. (They are to hold that candle in their hands till the end of the ceremony).
- Place the flower crown on her head and say—'Today, you are crowned as a woman. Now that you have begun your moon-time you are welcomed into the Circle of Women'. (The witnesses can then say together, Welcome Sister.)
- Present her with her token and say—'May this … give you strength and courage as you become a woman. May it remind you of this day as you were held in love and the highest regard by the Circle of Women'.
- Give her a heartfelt hug. Repeat for all participants.

Now let's sit down in the circle. Let everyone sit on the floor (or chairs if they are available). Now listen to the voices of the future. This moment is for you.

- Read the letters, one at a time. Read them slowly, mindfully. Put love and care in each word. Hold them through your reading in the highest regard. After each letter, ask everyone to take a couple of deep breaths to accept the words heard and to make space for the next letter. So, everything can be properly absorbed and welcomed.

- When you finish reading all the letters ask everyone to stand up.
- Say: 'I welcome you into the sisterhood of women. You will walk this path in joy, in sorrow, in pain, but also in love and in incredible happiness. Welcome my daughters, my sisters, my kin'.
- If you have prepared any poetry, read it now.
- Ask participants: 'Is there anything any of you would like to share with the circle or feel the need to say?'
- Allow the voices of the Maidens.
- Now the time has come to come back to our own time. In a clockwise direction walk back to the present. And as you are walking feel the years coming back filling you with wisdom and knowledge. Feel your body growing, and changing. Feel your flow coming and going allowing to you mature in your blood wisdom. Come back to here and now of today.
- When you have arrived in today, welcome everybody back. Thank them for their participation in the ceremony. Ask all the women to blow out their red candles.
- Go to the altar and blow out first the red candle and then the white one.
- Finish by saying—'So may it be and so it is'.
- Allow both circles to mingle, cuddle, laugh, cry. Have a feast together. Be sisters to one another.

Hopefully, this is the beginning of a beautiful and supportive women's circle.

The Young Goddess

A Maiden Goddess also known as a Virgin Goddess presides over spring, the waxing moon, and the rising energy of your menstrual cycle. Your bleed has just finished, your body is renewed, and your young new cycle has just begun. Young Goddess is a bringer of new beginnings, dawn, youth, passion, fresh potential, art, creativity, self-expression, beauty, intelligence, and skill. The Maiden represents purity and the innocence of childhood, where the soul can soar on the wings of her dreams, magic still exists, and makes believe still prevails. The Maiden reminds us to look after this magical child that lies within us. She reminds us to stay in touch with the childhood intuition and fantasies that are fuelling our dreams. She is bringing with her this incredible belief and hope that everything is possible and that we can achieve it all. Maiden doesn't know her sexuality yet but can feel the tiny pulls from her body, the awakening, the pre-flavour of what is to come. She doesn't treat it seriously though; she is all for playfulness and discovery. The world is her playground. She is brave and forthcoming. The Maiden is a discoverer. She discovers her body for the very first time. How does it feel when I'm touched in different places? What do I look like? She is curious and she is not tainted with the shadow of shame yet. If shame and discomfort with your body are present, connect to the Young Goddess within. Allow her to explore all the nooks and curves of your body. Do it slowly, without rushing. You are not touching yourself to gain pleasure, not yet. You are doing it to discover yourself, to see how different types of touch can feel. Try to look at yourself with fresh eyes—not one's weight heavily with the modern so-called 'canons of beauty'—find your own canons.

Why would you let others dictate to you what is and is not beautiful? You are the creatrix of your own reality—it's time we claim our rightful place in it. A place of beautiful natural females. Women that are not scared of ageing and curves. Women that are strong within their bodies. It all starts with the Maiden. Teach yourself how to see that world for the very first time and inhabit it with wholeness, courage, and strength. The Maiden is exploring the first stages of intimacy. We cannot hope to be intimate with each other without being truly intimate with ourselves first. How can you show your lover what brings you pleasure if you yourself have no idea of that? If your body hasn't been claimed by you yet. How can you give in to pleasure if you are too busy thinking how ugly or fat you may be? How can you truly feel your body if you constantly remain in your head? The Maiden can help you with that. Through the medium of touch the Young Goddess inserts this curiosity into your Yoni, learning and mapping all this previously undiscovered land. Because of the fear that patriarchy bestowed within us, we believed for long enough that masturbation comes from the devil's book. But what it is truly? It is self-discovery, self-love, self-compassion, and self-healing. And nothing about it is evil and dirty. And Maiden in her curiosity, openness, freshness, and dare can teach you all of that.

Your Maiden phase will feel different in May and different in October. It will vary depending on the moon and if she is waxing or waning. Open yourself to all those experiences, they are here to show you how you are truly feeling underneath all the pretences of everyday life and social expectations. They will show you where you are on your spiral journey and what path lies ahead.

If you ignore the Maiden coming through, if you try to silence her, you may find yourself in front of a tantrum. The unexpressed and not processed or listened to anger may overflow, making it a hard transition into your next phase. The new and fresh ideas will fall like last year's leaves to the ground and will burn in envy and jealousy of others. You will see them gone unfulfilled, and you may surrender to sadness. But youth need compassion and patience, and you can grant yourself both of those feelings. You can always slow down, observe what is happening within and remember. You can transition into the next phase wiser and make sure that in your new cycle the Maiden is not only noticed but also given her voice and expression. And this is the true power of your menstrual cycle. Nothing is finite or lost. Your whole life is filled with infinite possibilities and healing.

The Maiden opens herself to the direction of the East. And the East is the direction of new beginnings, of dawn, of new possibilities, of breath and air. Our menstrual cycle opens for us a new chapter and new possibilities each month. And each month we face the East with renewed hope and opportunity. Each cycle we can change and improve things that didn't work for us in the previous one. Each cycle we can refine our lives, we can boost our energy levels, and our creativity, and come back to the places that still need a little bit of work or processing. And each cycle we have an opportunity to know our Maiden a little bit better. We can give her more space to breathe and to explore. More space to become and to take us home to ourselves.

CHAPTER 6

Dancing with goddesses: Maiden unleashed

Artemis/Diana

In ancient Greek mythology, Artemis was the Virgin Goddess of the moon and night, hunting, the wilderness, wild animals, nature, vegetation, childbirth, care of children, and chastity. Diana was her Roman equivalent. Artemis has come to represent the variable energies of the feminine psyche. In Greek mythology, Artemis is the daughter of Zeus and Leto and the twin sister of Apollo. Artemis was born first, and legend has it she then assisted her mother in the birth of her brother. Artemis preferred to remain a Maiden goddess and had sworn never to marry. Similarly, to Artemis, Diana was born fully grown and was said to be tall and beautiful. Both were represented in art as wearing a quiver of arrows on their shoulders and holding a bow. Often accompanied by maidens, deer, and hounds. While Diana was a symbol of purity, she was often prayed to by women who wanted to conceive and by those already pregnant who were hoping for an easy birth. Both Artemis and Diana were praised for their intelligence. But like all goddesses, they both also had unpredictable natures and could be vengeful.

Both Artemis and Diana reveal physical strength and athleticism. They also rely on themselves and other women—their maidens, and this is a very important lesson for women today. We are living in a world that doesn't know the meaning of sisterhood anymore. Women are very harsh towards one another and very often we judge ourselves in a much more cruel way than we would ever judge a man. We are in constant rivalry and think we must flatten any female competition. Women are often scared of other women and the relationships between all of us is a thin thread. This suits the patriarchy immensely. If we could just come together, support ourselves, and have each other's back—our lives would be much easier, and we could return to the true meaning of the word 'sisterhood'. We can ask Artemis and Diana for help in this endeavour. Many of the goddess's rituals encouraged girls and women to come together and dance wildly in the light of the full moon. When women came together, there was no shame or embarrassment, there was an acceptance of the female body and its beauty. There was permission for self-discovery, wildness, and ecstasy. Because when women come together all is possible and magic happens. As sisters, we can spread love. To do that we must learn how to connect to the essence of the joyful heart and laughter, and this will release our power into motion.

Questions to journal with

- What does connecting to the Maiden archetype mean for me?
- Who am I as the Maiden today?
- How does the Maiden show herself in my life?
- How does the Meiden show herself in my menstrual cycle?
- What memories from my childhood does the Maiden bring forth?
- How can I find more Maiden energy in my life?
- How can I see my body through the eyes of the Meiden?
- Do I have enough joy and laughter in my life?
- How can I cultivate more joy and laughter every day?
- How can I celebrate the Maiden within?

Sacred gathering

It's time to gather your sisters together. Would you like to belong to a Sacred Moon Lodge, a Red Tent, a Sacred Gathering of Women who would come together once a month to laugh, cry, bleed, birth, die, and be re-born? To share stories of the past and create the way of the future. Gathering is deeply embedded in our DNA. We've always done it.

In times past women would go together into the land gathering food, while men would go hunting. Then they would bring the gathered supplies into the settlement and together they would work on cooking and preserving the rest for later. While working they would sing, tell stories, laugh, and tell jokes that made men blush, being together in a community. During their moon-time, they would gather in Red Tents or Moon Lodges spending time together, supporting one another, listening to one another, and creating not only community but also weaving the sisterhood. Sisterhood in which the blood bond had an entirely new meaning. Because you don't have to come from the same family to be someone's sister. You don't have to come from the same mother to be blood-bound to another woman.

Isn't that beautiful? In the past time when a woman in community would give birth, the rest of the women would come together to help feed her and her family, to clean and support her. We are not born to lead a solitary life, we thrive in community, but sadly we have forgotten this wisdom. Nowadays, so many women are struggling in solitude. We are experiencing an epidemic of loneliness. And each of us locked in the four walls of our houses, experiences anxiety, fear, and depression. And we give birth to our children alone, and must raise them up individually. And we bleed alone, in secrecy and shame. And behind a quiet wall, there is another woman experiencing the same horrors, and then another and another. And the magic disappears because in loneliness and sadness we forget the extent of our power. So, let's break that cycle. Let's get together. Let's create a community of sisters, supporters, friends, and maidens. Let's once again laugh together, cry together, and be together.

Create your own Sacred Gathering. Think of women you would like to invite and ask them if they know someone who may be interested too. It doesn't have to be a big group. It can start with you and one other woman only. You can set the intention that you would like it to grow, or it can remain intimate and cosy. You are the creatrix. What type of gathering would you like to be a part of? If you wish to work with Artemis or Diana, you can always ask for their help in creating the gathering of your maidens. But don't let the word maiden narrow you in inviting only women the same age. Open yourself to a diversity of ages. Ask your elderly neighbour if she would like to join. Or maybe your friend's daughter. Think about the architecture of your group. Would you like an open group, so new members will be able to join at any time? Or would you rather your group be closed and always meeting in the same format? What would you feel most comfortable with? Now think when you would like to meet—on a new moon, full moon, the first weekend of each month, or maybe the last one. Think where you would like to meet. Would you like to host it in your home? Maybe each meeting could be hosted by a different participant. Or maybe you prefer to put money together and rent a space in a village hall or your local school? Wherever you decide to have your meeting make sure the space is created with love and thought. You can introduce a seasonal theme and create a beautiful altar/centrepiece honouring the seasons or deities you are working with. The centrepiece can be in honour of femininity, sisterhood, or seasonal holidays.

You can ask everyone to bring something meaningful for them to put on the altar. You could ask everyone to bring cushions, blankets, and chairs, so everyone is comfortable. You could ask everyone to bring some food to share. You can find topics or rituals you would like to do together, you can watch a film, listen to poetry, and the possibilities are infinite. You can ask that each gathering be prepared by a different participant. Be curious, play, explore. The most important thing is that you would come together regularly, sharing, and supporting each other, that you create a bond. And that you know that whenever you are in need you can reach out to your sisters, and whenever they are, they can reach out to you. And you make yourself available and present, but you also put in place healthy boundaries.

If creating a Sacred Gathering is too much for you at this moment in time, check the internet for the local groups and meetings. Maybe something like that already operates in your neighbourhood and you will be able to join.

From my own experience, I can tell you that I cannot now imagine living a sister-less life. I'm lucky to have a beautiful biological sister, but also additionally Moon Sisters. I met my Moon Sister Isha when we were doing a Womb Medicine Woman Training. We were paired together to connect each week, to check in, to share and to support each other on our training journey. We were supposed to do it for a month. We never stopped. Now, a few years down the line we still meet weekly or fortnightly, and we share with each other the most intimate places in our lives. We trust each other, we raise each other up, we cry together, we laugh together, and the bond we share is not only deep but also sacred. In the past year we created, with another Moon Sister, Jamie, a beautiful Womb Healing Council where the three of us can meet monthly, holding space for each other, for our ups and downs in our therapy work and in personal lives, and the support we give to each other has changed my life. With my Moon Sisters, I truly understood what it means to be a woman. What it means to share, to be, to create together. How much we have changed our own worlds and through that how much the outside world has changed as well. And although we live in different countries, on different continents even, and we've never met in person (yet), our bond is not only true—it is magic.

So, my soul is calling your soul to the Sacred Gathering of Women.

The gift from my tribe

As an offering to you all and a beautiful contribution, I would like to share with you the wisdom of my Moon Sisters. I invited them to gift you on the pages of this book one of the practices they use in their womb-work. And here is the result of my request. Enjoy.

The gift from Jamie Wiggins

Return to the Garden. Tree of Wisdom meditation

Let us rewrite her-story together. You have entered a lush garden and approached a great-grandmother tree. She seems to slightly bend her branches to you and offers you a ripe and delicious peach. You take the fruit, warm, fuzzy, and heavy in your hand; its soft orange and crimson tones look like a sunset. You smell it. The scent is intoxicating, heady, and makes your mouth water. You take it to your mouth and sink your teeth in. The experience of the fruit fills all of your senses. The skin crunches in your mouth, the pulp is soft and squishy, and the flavour fills your mouth and nose with ecstatic rapture that you may have entirely forgotten existed. You have tasted the forbidden fruit. You have opened to your birthright as a cyclical human and opened to the wisdom of pleasure through all of your senses. This belongs to you, and you to it. You feel in your cells the cycle of creation. You know life and death as the sisters that they are. Welcome back to the garden.

Meditation

Find yourself in a comfortable seat at the base of the magnificent peach tree that has shared her wisdom with you. Find a soft and comfortable seat in her roots. She welcomes you in. You feel safe and held. You sit with her for as long as feels comfortable. Let your breath rise from the roots of the tree through your root to the top of your head. Repeat that cycle for at least one minute. Then on your next in-breath draw your breath from the centre of the Earth where the tree draws her own life force. Draw your breath up through your roots into your womb space. Repeat this cycle at least five times. Let the energy circulate in your womb space. Hold it there. What do you feel? Is it pulsing? Radiating? Is it quiet? Electric? There is no right answer. Now from this place filled with the delicious life force you have cultivated, plant the pit from your peach. Plant it deep in rich soil. Keep breathing from the centre of the Earth up into your womb. With each breath, your tree begins to grow. First, the roots begin to spiral deep down into the earth. Watch them grow. Then a small sprout pokes above the rich soil. Keep breathing from the centre of the Earth. You are now connected to the Earth through the tree of wisdom growing in your womb. Keep breathing from the heart of Gaia.

The energy is pulsing now as the tree grows taller. She is a sapling now. She is pulsing with the life force you have cultivated. She is gifting you with remembering your unshakeable source of wisdom. Let the roots grow deeper. As they grow deeper, they glow golden then the beautiful tree starts to stretch her branches out towards the sun. Arms unfurling. You watch her grow bountiful leaves, blossom through spring, grow heavy with fruit in the summer and as the leaves grow dry and deep purple fall back to the Earth in autumn. You wonder at her delicate beauty, standing naked and strong in the winter snow. You feel her alive in you. You see a cup in your hands. It is filled with your menstrual blood. You smile at this remembering. You pour your blood as an offering onto the roots of this sacred tree. You thank her for gifting you with her wisdom through each season, and each transition. You feel rooted in an unshakeable wisdom you always vaguely remembered but your conscious mind did not believe in. You rest in her presence. You breathe one last breath from the centre of the Earth up through the tree's roots, your root, your womb, the fertile ground she grows, through her trunk and outstretched branches. You let her essence radiate through your whole being. She is so happy you have found her. She wants you to know that her wisdom is always a breath away. Stretch your arms up like the branches of a tree. Open your eyes and move freely. Let the wisdom of your birthright fill your day.

The gift from Isha (Linda Isha Fitzwilliam)

Womb song

Allow yourself a time of rest.

Breathe into your womb.

Connect with your womb as a living resonance in you.

Notice the quality of your womb in this moment.

Allow that to be fully okay.

From your womb, as a body of resonance, let sound happen naturally.

Find the tone of voice which matches your womb's quality this moment.

Let your body emit vocal sounding (humming, toning) which is rooted in your womb.

Bathe in your sounding vibration.

After a while you may notice a difference in the tone of voice. Maybe your womb sounds change quickly. Let yourself be organically guided by your natural womb sound impulses.

Enjoy singing and listening to your own unique womb song.

When you feel guided to, slowly sink into silence.

Bathe in silence.

Notice the sensations in your womb, pelvis, spine, your heart, your whole body, and your energy field.

Give thanks to yourself for offering yourself time to attune deeply.

Effect: this practice supports the intimacy with your womb. The sound vibration can bring a healing effect to your womb, your cycle, your hormonal balance, your pelvic floor, and your overall emotional state. This practice offers relief during the premenstrual phase and supports an easy flow during your period.

You can do this practice every day, or during full moon and new moon times, or whenever you feel guided to.

Cordelia

This Celtic fairy goddess helps watch over the flowers that bloom in the springtime and summertime. She brings beauty into our lives along with the positive energies of the spring. Her main themes are prayer, beauty, fairies, and wishes. Her symbols are flowers and water. She helps with celebration, courage, gardening, flowers, joy, life changes, and stress management. Her stones are carnelian and citrine. As she is a water goddess one of her attributes is a well. Well-dressing festivals go back to ancient times. People believed that sacred wells held within them beneficial spirits. One could petition those spirits and as an offering people decorated the wells with Cordelia's symbols—garlands of spring flowers. The festival held in her honour was Beltane—the first day of summer. The Maiden Cordelia was celebrated for her virgin or flower aspect, she was a harbinger of the fruit to come. She was the daughter of the sea god, Lir, and was born as a sea goddess.

Today we can call upon Cordelia whenever we feel stressed or trapped indoors. We can close our eyes and visualise ourselves standing in the fields of flowers—free, courageous, and calm.

Questions to journal with

- How can I connect more with Nature?
- What benefits me from time in Nature?
- What can I do to improve my natural environment?
- What is my sacred space in Nature? (If you don't have one yet, could you go on the journey of finding one?)
- How do I tend my inner wells? (Inner wells of love, inspiration, creativity, energy, compassion?)

As Cordelia allows us to look deeply into the well within and the well without, I would like to invite you into this goddess's practice of looking deeply within the well of your beautiful *Yoni*. I would like to invite you to see the beauty reflected in you through the mirror of your *Yoni*. Can you dive deep within? Can you lose yourself in your own beauty? Can you adore and worship yourself? Can you see how truly beautiful you are? I can see you. I see your beauty. I can see this amazing goddess that you are.

Yoni *gazing practice*

For this practice, you will need a mirror and a comfortable space where you can remain undisturbed. You will also need time, as you don't want to be rushed or hurried. You can do this practice naked, but if you find this too cold, or your nakedness is not comfortable to you yet, that's okay. Put on a lovely dress you can easily lift, but don't put on any underwear. I would like you to feel comfortable and relaxed. Remember, this is your body and your practice. Make the space surrounding you a sacred space. Make it beautiful. Play your favourite music, light some candles, smudge or light some incense. If you prefer wax melts instead of incense that would be perfect too. Make your surroundings your own and make it special. You can do this practice on your bed, on the chair, or on the floor. How do you feel today? What do you prefer? Bring cushions and blankets. You are the queen of comfort, go for it fully. Are you ready? When you are, rest comfortably on the cushions. Allow them to prop you up, so you can easily move, but also stay in that position for some time. Make sure your neck is supported, so you won't strain any muscles. In this supported position, be it on your bed, chair, or on the floor, look down at your body. Look at yourself with love and curiosity, as if you were looking for the very first time. See the curve of your breasts and if you are naked the shape of your nipples. See the outline of your tummy, the shape of your hips, your pubic bone, maybe pubic hair, and your amazing, strong legs. Look at your beautiful vessel. Your body is the temple of your spirit. Look how beautiful you are. Breathe deeply and fully. When you are ready, take the mirror in your hand and allow your legs to open. If you feel strong resistance to opening your legs, that's okay, respect that and respect the needs of your body—just look at your beautiful shape and stay present with yourself. You can repeat this practice as many times as you need until you are ready to move it further.

If you feel your legs opening with ease, allow them to do so. Open your legs and support them on cushions, so you can still be comfortable and relaxed. Lower the mirror in between your legs, so you have the full view of your beautiful *Yoni*. Here she is. Look at her beauty and uniqueness. Although we are all women, we are also all different and all beautiful in our uniqueness. Look at your labia majora and labia minora, at your clitoral hood, the perineum strip. Look at the way your beautiful *Yoni* opens and closes with each move you are making. Is she moist or dry today? What colour dominates today? Does she feel sore or timid, or maybe open and soft? There is no right or wrong way of doing this practice. There is no right or wrong in the way your *Yoni* will look like. This is the gate to your womb—the first gate to your feminine power. Look at your beautiful *Yoni* and see her truly. Acknowledge her—I see you. And I see myself. In my beauty, in my uniqueness, in my perfection. This is what I look like. And if you wear the scars on your *Yoni*—the physical or the emotional ones (maybe after birthing your babies, or maybe after the sexual assault), look at them now with love and compassion. This is what I look like today, and the map on my Yoni shows the courage and immense strength I possess. My beautiful *Yoni* is the well of possibilities. This is the well of healing. This is also the well of love and pleasure. Allow yourself to gaze at your beautiful *Yoni* with respect, love, compassion, and curiosity. Gaze at her for as long as you wish to and for as long as it feels comfortable. Repeat this practice as often as you please. Gaze at your *Yoni* at different moments of your cycle. Notice how she is changing, how you are changing.

If you would like to take this practice deeper—bring to your *Yoni* gazing session a notepad and pencils or crayons. Place your mirror in a way that will free your hands but will allow you to see her and draw what you see. In your picture, you can dress her in flowers or stars, and allow your inspiration to flow. See your *Yoni* fully in her beauty and allow it to come through in your picture. By allowing yourself to see your *Yoni* properly, without any agenda, without needing her to look in a certain way or perform certain things. When you just allow yourself to see her for what she is, to see her in her beauty, a deep healing happens. Healing and acceptance. And this is the first step to accepting yourself, a gift of love that must start with the 'I'. That must come from you first before you can expect it to come from the other. And this is the first step to embodying your feminine power. The first step to understanding your own divinity. You are a goddess. I can see you. Now is the time for you to see yourself too.

Idunn

Idunn, also spelt Idun, or Iduna, in Norse mythology is the goddess of spring and rejuvenation and is the wife of Bragi, the god of poetry. The goddess was renowned for her youthful beauty. She was the keeper of the magic apples of immortality, which the gods must eat to preserve their youth. She was growing them in her enchanted western garden named Appleland. In the stories of King Arthur, Appleland was called Avalon. As the keeper of the golden apples, the goddess was responsible for the well-being of all the Norse gods.

In the Christian tradition, the apple was significant for the fall of man. That was the fruit from the Tree of Knowledge. Tasting it led to the first parents being expelled from the Garden. It also led to the 'menstrual curse'. The Norse people considered apples sacred and essential for the continuation and extension of life. Associated with resurrection, containers of these sacred fruits were placed in graves—to nurture the souls of the mortals as they travelled from one life to the next, from one world to the next. The Norse also believed that the soul could be passed from body to body, contained within the flesh of the apple, making it not only the fruit of knowledge but also a keeper of the human soul.

Idunn was the goddess of magic, immortality, and time. She represents the Earth's seasons. Following the story from *Goddesses in World Mythology*, Idunn was the keeper of the golden apples that made the gods immortal. One day Loki was snatched by an eagle and dragged across the ground for miles and miles. The eagle agreed to let Loki go if he promised to bring Idunn into the world of men. Loki convinced Idunn that he had found a tree that grew golden apples just like hers, so she went with him to see it. The eagle was waiting and swooped down snatching Idunn and carrying her and her apples to the land of the giants. The eagle was the giant Thiazi, who wanted the gods to age while he remained young. As the gods aged and became weaker, they began searching for Idunn. They discovered that she had left with Loki, so he was summoned and told to bring her back. Loki asked for Freyja's falcon skin and flew to the giant's land. He found Idunn and changed her into a nut, flying with her in his claws back to Asgard, returning the god's immortality and strength.

Idunn with other goddesses created the Asynjur, the judicial community that holds daily councils with other deities. That made her also the goddess of justice and one of the supreme beings. She is associated as well with love, divination, and dreams.

The Maiden archetype represents purity and the innocence of childhood, where the soul's dreams and magic are still very much alive. But there is also a darker side to our Maiden. Shadow Maiden is very self-centred, and all her dreams and energy are expended on achieving her own personal needs and goals. She forgets to look after the magical child that dwells within us all. She asks you to look at your selfish dreams and aspirations and take no account of the needs of others. The Shadow Maiden is part of the Maiden archetype, and we must acknowledge her and bring her into balance with the Maiden-self—so we can find the right balance in life. So let us feed some apples to our Shadow Maiden. Let us bring her some light.

In practice with Idunn, I would like to invite you to travel through the portal of your womb into your Maiden-self. To look into the surface of the well and be able to see through time and space. Idunn is the goddess of time, magic and dreams and she can help us with that. When approaching this practice, you can acknowledge Idunn in her divinity, if you wish so. You can create an altar for her, offering flowers and apples and maybe putting on it a picture from when you were young. Light some white candles. You can write an invocation to the goddess stating your intention for your work. Your intention is to meet with your Maiden-self and with your Shadow Maiden and hear their message. To open yourself to the essence of the Maiden imprint in your cells and through acknowledging her, listening to her, and letting go of things that need letting go of, heal your present self. Remember to have safety measures in place—a therapist, a family member you can talk to, or a women's group to process the messages that will come up. Get your journal ready, burn some incense, and create a sacred space. Even if you decide not to work with Idunn, create that sacred space for yourself and for your Meiden-self. You are going to connect with your Sacred Feminine, with your sacred divinity—acknowledge that for yourself. Embrace her. Are you ready?

Connecting to your Maiden-self meditation

Create your sacred space

Lie or sit down comfortably. Breathe easily and gently—in through your nose and out through your nose or mouth—you choose. How would you like to breathe today? Notice the cold air coming in through your nose, the air is warming up inside of your body and then the warm air is coming out of your mouth (or nose). Breathe like that for a moment, in and out, gently, naturally. Notice that with each breath your breathing is becoming slower and deeper, and that with each breath your body is becoming more and more relaxed. Now I would like to invite you to begin the wave breath. On the in-breath take the energy and the breath from the bottom of your feet and allow it to travel up your body to the top of your head. On a gentle pause between in-breath and out-breath, allow this energy to linger at the top of your head, and then on the out-breath flow the energy and the breath down your body to your feet. In and up, out and down. Breathe like that for a few in-breaths and out-breaths. Now, if you are ready, please place your hands on your womb. On the in-breath allow the breath and the energy to travel up to the top of your head, pause there for a second and on the out-breath allow it to slowly flow into your womb space. Slowly and gently, through your throat, through your heart—your mighty drum, right down into your womb space. Take as much time as you need. Breathe deeply in and out of your womb space. Allow the life-giving force of your breath to enter your womb. Breathe fully into your womb space.

You are in your womb space now. How does it feel to be there today? Can you see lights or colours? What language is your beautiful womb speaking to you today? Breathe deeply into your womb space. Looking down you can see a sheet of water. You can feel a very strong pull towards it. Let go of all resistance and allow the pull to take you into this beautiful well. Let go and submerge into this amazing pool of water. Go through it like through a magical gate. On the other side, there is a beautiful grove filled with trees and spring flowers. Take in your surroundings. Where are you? What does this place look like? Can you feel the grass underneath your feet? Experience everything fully. Give yourself time. Breathe deeply. You can see from the little woods up ahead a beautiful maiden approaching. Look at her. What does she look like? She approaches you and takes your hand in hers. The touch is warm and welcoming. You feel like coming back home. The Maiden looks into your eyes and starts talking. She knows you so well and tells you the story of who you are. What is she telling you? Listen. Open yourself to whatever comes. Feel self-love and self-worth emanating from her. Feel those feelings starting to grow within you now as well. She smiles at you and beckons you to follow her. Hand in hand you are allowing her to lead you. You walk together through a beautiful meadow until you reach a little pond. You kneel at the pond and look in. To your surprise, you cannot see your reflection. Instead of seeing yourself and the Maiden reflected on the water's surface, you can see a different Maiden. She looks darker and not so happy. This is your Shadow Maiden. Look into her eyes and allow her to speak. Hear what she has to say. What happened to her? How can you help her? How can you embrace her? Allow her to voice her needs. Listen. Breathe deeply. When she finished talking, tell her you love her. Tell her now.

As you are saying and meaning these beautiful words, you can see the Maiden next to you reaching her hand into the water. The Shadow Maiden reaches her hand out to her too and when their touch meets, the Shadow Maiden is absorbed into her light counterpart. Now your Maiden-self is complete again. Filled with her light and her shadow in perfect balance. 'Now you are complete as well', says the Maiden and takes your hands in hers. You feel an immense warmth and tingling. You close your eyes and feel your Maiden-self merging into you. 'Welcome home, sister' you hear. You can truly feel all the lessons and messages of your Maiden-selves within you now. You feel accepted, loved, and whole again. It doesn't matter if there are still any unresolved issues left. The maidens who came to you today have been accepted and listened to and their lessons have been processed. You can feel it in your bones. You can feel it in your DNA. Allow the balancing force from this encounter to envelop you. Feel your growth. Feel yourself surrounded with love, acceptance, beauty, and curiosity. Feel parts of you coming back home. Thank them and welcome them back. This is your path to becoming whole once again. You are on the right track; you are walking this path now. Breathe deeply. Feel the Maiden-selves melting within you, soaking in. Let go of expectations. Just be with this beautiful experience. Breathe deeply.

Now the time has come to leave this beautiful meadow. Walk back to the pool and when you are ready submerge yourself into the water. Through the well of this beautiful warm water, you are travelling back into your womb space. Breathe deeply. You are back in your womb space now. Breathe deeply into your womb. Now I would like to invite you to gather all the energy, all the wisdom from your womb and on the in-breath move it up into your heart space. On the out-breath move it back to your womb. Move this beautiful energy to your heart so you can feel your truth. Now on the in-breath, let's move this energy to the top of our head. On the out-breath move it back into your womb. Move this beautiful energy to the top of your head, so you can know and remember your truth. Now on the in-breath, move this energy to the top of your head and on the out-breath move it down all over your body. Surround yourself with this energy like in a cocoon. Allow its medicine to penetrate you, and let it go. Let it flow where it wishes to. If this energy wishes to flow into your body, let it be so. If into Mother Earth, allow it to be so. If it spreads and flows into the world or disappears, just let it go. Gently, easily, and with trust. Breathe normally. Slowly bring yourself back. Introduce gentle movement into your fingers and toes. Stretch your arms and legs. Gently move and stretch your neck. And when you are ready, but only when you are ready, open your eyes. You are fully present, safe and at peace. You feel loved and complete.

You can now write about your experience in your journal. Draw, paint, and express your experience in a creative way. This is how you acknowledge what has happened. This is how you bring it to the material realm, how you can process it and let it go.

If you feel in any way triggered, please make sure that you are safe. Reach out to your friend, therapist, or women's group and process this experience with them. It is very important you do so. This is a part of your healing journey, a very important part.

You can visit your Maiden-self whenever you feel the need. You can slowly work through things from your past through the magic and power of your womb. And remember, your Maiden-self is an important part of you, and she has many lessons to teach you. Open yourself to her wisdom. Allow her in. Befriend her. She is an integral part of you, a very important one. Let her in. Merge with her. Become whole once more.

PART 3

JOURNEY FROM LOVER TO MOTHER

CHAPTER 7

Breast wisdom

Women's sexual health is rooted in Judeo-Christianity and shrouded in shame. In our culture, we seem to have two main archetypes—that of the Mother and that of the Whore—and sadly there is this great void in between with nothing that we, as women, could reference to. The Mother should stay hidden in the house, the image of the Whore can be abused on the streets. Sexualisation of women's breasts came together with the desecration of the goddess, when patriarchy rose to power. Only then did the breasts become objectified. To be honest, this sexualisation and objectification happened not only to our breasts but to the whole woman's body. Pornography has become the wound of the world we are living in. A bleeding and gnawing wound with no possibility of healing. But when you think about it, the breast is a representation of the divine, of creation, of sustainability and of safety.

Breasts symbolise life, fertility, nourishment, and holy femininity. Breasts used to be worshipped as a life-giving force. Now they are the means of sexual satisfaction. It is fine to advertise sexual lingerie and exposed breasts and almost naked women to do so. It is fine to expose naked breasts in pornography. But in our society, it is still so much harder to stomach when women breastfeed in public. When the breast comes forth in its true meaning of life-giving sustenance, it is still a taboo. But when you think about it, children nursing at the breasts of their mothers are drinking the life itself, as no death has touched that drink. It is created by a living being and offered to another being and as such it becomes a part of life itself. Through milk, our first food, we gain an intimate connection with our mothers. This is a sacred act in itself. Isn't this miraculous and amazing? Isn't that beautiful? Well, I think so.

There are so many depictions of goddesses breastfeeding their off-spring and at the same time humanity. Goddesses Isis and Hathor were both milk goddesses and were connected to the Milky Way, which was considered to be the milk that flowed from the udders of a heavenly cow. For the ancient Egyptians, the image of the goddess Isis suck-ling her son Horus was a powerful symbol of re-birth. The importance of this holy act was transferred later to Rome, where the cult of the goddess was established. Breast milk in Egypt was so much more than an earthly substance. The hieroglyphs depict kings drinking the milk of the Holy Mother. This gave them longevity, vitality, and divinity. Milk is magic. Milk was also used in healing.

The 'milk of a woman who has born a son' was a common ingredi-ent in Egyptian medicine and in magical spell recipes. Another dairy deity was Iat. From the hieroglyphic descriptions in Pyramid texts, we learn that a 'milky drink' was part of sacrifice rituals used to prepare the offerings table, and that the 'sacred milk' was also used to treat asthma, and many more complaints. Milk also had an association with the Other World. The Pharaoh after death would receive new life from Hathor's milk on his journey to the Other World. In Christian iconog-raphy, the Nursing Madonna shows the Virgin Mary breastfeeding the infant Jesus. However, the symbolism of breastmilk went much further in Christian iconography. It is not unusual to see the image of the Virgin Mary breastfeeding a saint (for example, St Bernard of Clairvaux). In medieval times breastfeeding was a common fact of life. It was associ-ated with being fed not only physically but also spiritually. Having a depiction of the Virgin Mary exposing her breast and feeding faithful saints was not considered scandalous but was meant to signify a deeper spiritual reality. It was the highest of blessings.

It was giving a gift of oneself. So, what has happened to the breast? Why has it fallen from the highest of heavens to the lowest of hells? Why are we still allowing that to happen? We were told that our breasts were too small, too big, too different, and not beautiful. We were also told that about our entire bodies. And we believed. And we are allowed to be persuaded to chase after the cannon of beauty dictated to us by the patriarchy. We allowed the scalpels of so-called beauty to give us different shapes and sizes, so we were able to catch up to the desires of men and pornography; to the God of Mammon. And by doing that the health of breasts across the entire world suffered. Statistics show that many women across the world will develop breast cysts in their lifetime. Some will be benign, but some will progress into more sinister outcomes. Breast cancer is the most common cancer there is. Following the Global Breast Cancer Statistics, (www.breastcanceruk.org.uk) we read that in:

> 2020, 11.7% of all cancers diagnosed were female breast cancer. In 2020, there were 2.26 million women diagnosed with breast cancer and 685.000 deaths globally. As of the end of 2020, there were 7.8 million women alive who were diagnosed with breast cancer over the past 5 years. In 2019, there were 25.100 men diagnosed with breast cancer and 12.100 deaths globally.

Numbers don't lie. The desecration of Gaia, of the goddess, is also a desecration of women, but with a dire consequence for all of us. We were told that dysregulation in our body is the fault of our genetics. Sometimes it is, but not always. Sadly, we are living in a very toxic world (emotionally and physically). The trauma of living here is also filled with toxins. Sexual violence, domestic abuse, and desecration of women's bodies are present all over the world. We are told that others know our bodies better than we do. That we have no idea. But that is the biggest lie we have been told. No one knows our bodies as well as we do. We forgot how to create a partnership between ourselves and our bodies, but this is a vital lesson. We must stay steadfast to what we know is true because we can feel it. We must learn how to trust ourselves, our bodies, and our truths. It is a revolutionary act to listen to your body. It is a sacred language that we must remember how to decode. But our culture is still trying so hard to tell us otherwise. Please hear me now. Your endocrine system that governs your hormones is not your enemy.

We have been conditioned from a very young age to believe it to be true. There is a certain indoctrination to push us to believe that it is better for us to have fewer and fewer periods, how we can pretend that we don't bleed each month. Our hormones are connected to our Divine Feminine. They act as a powerful conduit of information and feedback.

They are guidance and warning systems, alerting us when we are not getting what we need for our health. We must turn back to Earth to help us heal. A return to the Earth, to Mother Gaia is a return to self. It is a lifesaving act. It will save us as a species. It will save humanity and our beautiful planet. It is time to give Gaia back her divinity. To see in her the goddess that she is.

Our breast holds a lot of emotion and emotional trauma. Just as the entirety of our body does. Being a Zero Balancing practitioner taught me that trauma is imprinted in our bones. Not only that, trauma hides in soft tissues too. Trauma imprints that have to do with the feminine will be stored in our feminine parts—our breasts and the womb. And right now, we carry not only our own trauma but also one from generations past. Unresolved trauma from our feminine line, from our ancestors. We have been taught to avoid pain at all costs. Therefore, we are trying so hard not to hear our bodies speaking to us. But there is so much wisdom in our bodies, if we only allow ourselves to believe in what we know is true. Bodies speak to us in a very subtle way. If we remain deaf, they will start screaming at us. Your body screams in pain. Pain is a language that we still are trying to suppress instead of getting to the root of it. Instead of opening our hearts and asking the most vital question: What are you trying to tell me? What is happening within? And then we listen. We listen with the wholeness of our being to that answer. And we nourish ourselves. The nourishment that we give to our bodies is also the nourishment that we should give ourselves, so we can mother ourselves. So, we can connect with this powerful archetype and use it as an act of self-love and self-care. By taking care of our own bodies, by mothering ourselves, we turn back to our beautiful planet and begin to love, respect, and heal her as well. We have this power within ourselves. We are Mother Gaia. We are the breasts of life itself. We are life-giving milk. We are.

So, let's get to know our bodies with respect, love, and compassion. Every day this alchemical treasure takes us through so much wonder and discovery. It's time to notice. It's time to pay attention. It's time to listen.

Breast self-examination

This is the practice I would like to invite you to make as a part of your cycle tracking, so you can know your breast intimately and truly. By checking your breast each cycle, you will get to know each tiny thickening of your tissue, each tiny lump. You will notice that hormonal changes associated with your menstrual cycle normally increase your breast lumpiness and swelling. And that is absolutely normal. The lumps will come and go and by knowing your body you can save yourself a lot of unnecessary stress. The best time to perform breast self-examination is a few days to a week after your menstrual flow ends. Try aiming for the same day (or three-day period) each cycle. Women using oral contraceptives are advised to perform their breast self-examination (BSE) each month on the day they begin a new packet of pills. When you are pregnant, you still should carry on with BSE. The best scenario would be if you could have an exam performed by your care provider at the onset of pregnancy, then repeated later in pregnancy and again postnatally. You yourself perform it every month of your pregnancy, noticing the changes, and giving yourself this beautiful self-care time.

I've learnt how to perform BSE and what to look out for from one of my herbal mentors, Aviva Romm. When doing BSE these are the breast changes and warning signs to look out for.

- A new lump or hard knot in the breast or armpit.
- A lump or thickening that does not decrease after menstruation.
- A change in the size, shape, or symmetry of the breast.
- Thickening, swelling, or indentation in the breast.
- Redness, or scaliness of the nipple or breast skin.
- Nipple discharge, especially if it's bloody, clear, or sticky and occurs without squeezing your nipple (please note that nipple discharge is usually normal in pregnancy).
- Nipple tenderness or pain.
- Nipple retraction.
- Any breast changes that concern you!

If the lumps are symmetric between both breasts, it is probably normal breast tissue. Questionable lumps are usually firm, irregular nodules that are fixed in place. They do not typically fluctuate in size with the menstrual cycle. Nipple discharge in most cases is caused by non-cancerous conditions, and less than 10% of nipple discharge is due to cancer. Nevertheless, it is imperative for you to notice and have it checked.

When checking your breasts, you can do it sitting or standing. Palpate gently around your breast and nipple. Squeeze your nipple gently and rub it between your fingers. Go all the way around your breast, then lift your arm and put your hand behind your head. Check your breast again, this time going also around the armpit area, the tissue between the breast and the armpit and next to your breast where you can feel the ribs on the side of it. Check everything gently with your fingers. Then repeat on the other breast. Feel yourself in this way. What does your breast tissue feel like? Is it comfortable to touch yourself in this way? Do you feel any type of blockages? Or maybe pain? This is all very important information for you. Make a note of it in your journal. When you do BSE during your next cycle, compare the notes. Are there any differences? How do you feel now? This is a guide to your health, your conversation with your body—notice as much as you can.

After you finish your BSE, you may choose to give yourself a loving breast massage. This is a beautiful path of self-love and self-attention. This is also a beautiful gratitude practice. A gratitude for the wonder that your body is. There are many ways you can massage your breasts. Just find a way right for you. Be intimate with your touch—what feels good for you right now. Do you prefer gentle strokes or maybe a stronger squeeze? Don't restrict your massage to BSE only. Do it throughout the month as often as possible, as often as you want to. You can massage your breast underneath the shower, or afterwards using oil. The oil I like to use for my breast massage is rosehip oil. Sometimes I will add to it a few drops of rose essential oil or frankincense oil (but always remember never to put essential oils on your skin undiluted). You can create your own essential oils compilation for your breast massage, but always choose gentle oils as breast tissue is very delicate. I found that rosehip oil does wonders for my breasts, and this massage always leaves me calm, relaxed and happy. I can't stress enough how important this relationship should be for every single woman.

CHAPTER 8

The juiciness of ovulation

Summertime

As spring unfolds her wings and departs, the warmth of the sun brings forth the summertime. And with the summer life begins once more. A life more mature but still fresh and filled with wonder. The Earth's rotational axis is tilted more toward the sun maximising the amount of light we are getting. The days are long, the weather is warm, and energy is abundant. Summer brings with it youth and vitality through this dynamic and abundant energy. But the quality of this energy is very different to the one we got to know during springtime. All our senses are almost in overdrive throughout long days, fresh warm air, vibrant colours, coolness of the water, smell of flowers and fresh grass. We feel energised, vigorous, adventurous, and ready to explore the world. But summer brings fort also this beautiful energy of coming of age and maturation. Unlike the spring when new life is gently coming forth, in summer everything is in full bloom. Fruit is ripe on trees, meadows are filled with flowers, and life is at its peak of the energy of expression. You can feel it in the air, feel it in your bones and become strong, healthy, and filled with beauty. The whole Earth is ready for love. For the embodiment of romance filled with mystery, excitement, and sex.

Summertime is the season of the light. The summer solstice marks the longest day of the year, giving the entire population of your city the greatest exposure to the sun. You can stay outside longer, and enjoy warmer nights and adventures. And with the abundance of the sun's rays, you can see more clearly—both physically and spiritually, as light is the symbol of both awareness and illumination. This is also the season when harvest is beginning to mature. It is a time to prosper, to explore, to go out and be in the world. It's a time of summer storms, sometimes violent, but mostly bringing relief and solace. When spring holds the promise, summer is ripe with its fulfilment.

The Lover and the power of ovulation

In each cycle, the day comes when the Maiden's *Yoni* mapping is almost complete. It shifts from the discovery of one's body to the discovery of pleasure. This is the moment when the Lover awakes. The Lover seeks passion. The Lover is awakened by the growing power—pre-ovulation and ovulation. Ovulation or your inner summer is the time of sensuality and sensual awakening. It is a magnetic time filled with attraction, generosity, flow, pleasure, charm, visibility, and mastery. The energy is at its highest and that drives forth optimism and love for others. You feel that you are fully out there in the world, conquering and winning all. Nothing is impossible. You can do anything that takes your fancy. You are at the top of your world. And like in the outer summer, this is the time of abundance and plenitude. There are no limits now. You are glowing with your inner-power and strength. You are the embodiment of the goddess herself. Everything seems easy. Whatever task you undertake flows wonderfully and with ease. Your creativity and self-expression are pouring through the pores of your skin. You are sure that life loves you and the universe has your back. If you've heard your calling and are true to yourself, this time can be truly magical, and you can feel that you are weaving with life itself. This is the perfect time to express yourself freely and truly. If you find a close connection with yourself and your cycle, summertime can be very grounding. If you skip the connection bit, you may lose your head, and put yourself in situations that are not desirable or even dangerous.

At this time your sexual energy is heightened and most of us can feel easily aroused. This sensation of rising sexual energy can be very strong and awe-inspiring. You may feel yourself charged up by the Earth's creative force. Everything around you become sexual. Eating, walking, dressing up—all are charged with this current of energy, this excitement and bliss. If you fight it, it will become overpowering and will break you down. If you give in to it, honouring your body and changes within, you can harness this energy towards your creative projects, life, and inspiration. This is a very potent time—rich and abundant. You are one with nature and you can bloom as beautifully as she is. In our culture, we are taught that sexuality is sinful. It is embarrassing and shouldn't be mentioned, especially not by women. It is something we can make dirty jokes about and keep under the duvet. But sexual energy is the energy of creation. It lies at the beginning of all things. If you open yourself to it and allow it to penetrate you, you can find a magnitude of healing within. But this energy is not only strong, but it is also raw. If there is a wounding in your Lover archetype, summertime may be very difficult and challenging. If you have experienced sexual trauma during the summer of your life, the rising energy may feel scary and not safe. If you have experienced body shaming, violence, bullying, relationship problems, difficult birth, self-esteem problems, anxiety, and stress, this beautiful time can be quite stormy for you. When dark clouds gather and cover the sun, the wind picks up and slashes through the city, lightning splits the heavens in half and thunder deafens us with its roar. When the sky opens in a violent cry, the accompanying energy is one of chaos. And chaos scares us terribly. Chaos is the opposite of order. And what are we craving more of in our lives than order? But chaos is also a part of the creative process. Creation comes from within chaos. So does healing. Therefore, cycle tracking is imperative. To notice, to observe, to be with the feelings, changes, difficulties, and to let them go, release them when the time is right. To discover what lies beneath and when it surfaces in our cycle is the first step to healing. It won't happen overnight. Sometimes it takes a few cycles to just simply notice the pattern, but that takes you one step closer to the summer of your dreams. To the whole of you.

The Lover energy, like every other archetype, is also affected by your approach to the entire cycle. If you haven't had time for proper wintering and used a lot of the energy in the phase when you were supposed to charge your batteries and rest. If you didn't allow your Maiden to explore and plant the seeds, the summer won't be filled with abundance. There will be no space for that nor energy. You will be spent already so early in your cycle. Your body won't have the strength to feel the sexual rise and you will feel tired, frustrated, and angry. How can you feel the pick in your energy, when your leaves have begun to fall already? These are the beautiful and very important lessons of cycle tracking. But don't despair. This is life and life is not perfect. Life is to be lived. To fall and to rise once more, to run, to stumble, to jump, to laugh and to cry. Life is chaos. Life is creation. And your cycles come and go in a spiral pattern. You can gather the information from each phase and change your approach to find healing. If you have spent yourself and your energy in winter and spring, rest in the summer so you will be able to discover and enjoy a beautiful golden autumn. And then make notes for the next cycle, so you can respect winter, appreciate the spring, and feel the summer's energy fully. Cycle tracking teaches us that nothing is constant and that nothing lasts forever. Everything passes and this situation shall pass too. Your trauma can be healed. You can be whole once more. You can break at some point again, but with the proper self-care put in place, putting yourself together again will happen faster and be less painful.

Summer can be a very transcendent and intoxicating energy and it is easy to become ungrounded and lose the connection to oneself. Our longing to be loved and accepted can drive us to do everything to fit in and not stand apart. But often we cannot remain forever as part of the group if we are to show our true selves honestly. And it can be truly challenging and scary. The pleasure of this time can keep us distant from the difficult parts of life. Because we feel so fabulous, we can become insensitive about the feelings of others. At this time, we feel tougher and this can bring us more distance to our own true feelings and needs. We become swept in the moment and taken with the current. The socialised self can come forth and overshadow the true you, showing only what you imagine is good about yourself and what society tells you is good. This can become a very big block to intimacy and can become a source of shame. There is a fine line between the freedom to feel this beautiful abundant joy and the slippery slope of hedonism and excess.

Summertime is juicy, and so is your body. You bite into the ripe fruit and feel the pleasure of sticky juice trickling down your hand. Your body is ripe as well, and the juices of your *Yoni* are dripping richly down your thighs. You are ready; you are awakened; the energy that has been rising since the beginning of this cycle has reached its peak. You are the Lover personified and you are ready to make love to the universe.

You can feel you are part of that universe with your entire being. You are fully present in your body and ready for waves of pleasure. You are alive, and you vibrate with this new and strong energy—you are the goddess of love. Nothing can stop you. Your entire body is breathing this energy with you. Breath after breath, pulse after pulse—you are at the top of the world. And then subtly the energy begins to shift once again. You begin to feel more grounded, and your body is responding differently. You also discover a different kind of love for yourself, and others, and you realise that the time of the Mother has come.

Journey from Lover to Mother

As the Lover is more focused on taking, the Mother is the giver. She is giving of herself, of your love and abilities, and she is fully conscious of your connection with Earth. She is filled with intelligence, wisdom, strength, and passion. She is caring, selfless, and nurturing. The Mother archetype is filled with vigour and energy, and she radiates love for the whole of creation. She is the creatrix, and she is fully conscious of her inner-power. This archetype balances the outward expression of energy with the inner expression of love and care. It can bring a feeling of satisfaction and wholeness, harmony and belonging. The Mother phase is deeply tangled with the Lover and begins when ovulation is fully established. It awakens the sense of self-confidence, and self-worth and is still very much facing outwards, towards others. The sex drive is still very strong, and the love for the partner is at its deepest. The care and love that you feel opens your awareness to the needs of your partner, but it can also open the awareness to your own needs. You can perceive him/her as your own child, but you can also reach deeply within and discover your own inner-child. With strong sexual energy, the creative energy becomes deep and rooted within your body and womb and strong and vivid dreams can open you to the world beyond.

But like everything in the universe, the Mother also has her dark side. There is the 'Good Mother' of nurturing, of the mysteries of birth, one who is holding, bearing, and releasing. But there is also the 'Terrible Mother', one who pushes away, tears, devours, and who is the mistress of the mysteries of death. They both have their own place in existence, and they are both equally important. Noticing them and working with them allows the healing to happen. Penelope Shuttle and Peter Redgrove sum it up delightfully in their book *The Wise Wound*.

> The Mother is concerned with the life and death of the ovum, she will bear if she can, and she will take into herself her dead offspring, which is her other side, the Terrible Mother. The Transformative Feminine is concerned, however, with spiritual children, which she will either bear, as the Muse, or destroy and reabsorb in the ecstasy of madness: it is her own transformation by which she transforms others—just as the Mother by her pregnancy and labour evolves the abilities of fatherhood in man.
>
> (p. 132)

Our whole cycle is transformative not only for ourselves but also for everyone who meets us—our friends, children, partners, and the whole world. They are influenced by each of our phases and each of our archetypes plays a role in their lives as well. When you think about it in this way, it's quite a responsibility, isn't it? Working with and understanding the cycle and phases we are going through stands at the foundation of a healthy society. I deeply believe that when we understand and heal women's bodies and cycles, we will be able to heal the Earth. I also believe that the answers to all the questions of the universe can be found in the female body. We just must stop and listen, with an open mind, curiosity and without judgement.

There may be many triggers present in your body and mind during the Mother phase. You may be triggered if your relationship with your own mother wasn't that good. It may affect you considering becoming the Mother yourself and bring forth deep wounding. But your Mother phase is incredibly healing. By tapping into your inner-mother, you can work on deep levels with your inner-child. You can support yourself in ways your own mother couldn't. You can hold and nurture yourself. You can see yourself in your childhood and as a grown woman and you can bridge them together. You have so much power and you can make yourself whole again. You don't need many external resources for that as true and deepest healing comes from within. It comes with permission, acceptance, and trust. If you grew up without a mother, or she wasn't as present as you needed her to be, you can give yourself this attention and comfort now. Through holding your inner-mother, you can heal your Maiden-self. Through meditation, journeying, journaling, through womb-work, you can bridge the time gap and become the mother you always needed and wanted. Through embodying your inner-mother, you can begin the journey of forgiveness.

You may find your Mother phase difficult and triggering if you experienced miscarriage. There may be fears surfacing during this phase, and your dream memories may be terrible and overwhelming. Often, you may not even realise what is triggering this bodily response. But if you ask yourself, have I permitted myself to truly grieve my lost baby? Have I released them yet? Or have I absorbed them fully and allowed the Terrible Mother to take control? Maybe the time has come to allow the Terrible Mother forth, and by working with her you will allow yourself to release all the energy that is holding you in grief and in the past. Remember that Terrible Mother is not evil. She is the polar opposite of the Good Mother and as an archetype is equally important. Acknowledging her and working with her will bring healing and solace as well. You may need a few cycles to accomplish that. You may need external help in the form of counselling or grief therapy. But healing is not a speedy affair. Healing is a process, healing is a journey, a lifetime adventure. Don't rush yourself, take each cycle as it comes. See what is surfacing and when, observe, make notes, and compare cycle to cycle. In the journey of your life, you are a constant observer and a witness. Begin witnessing now and see where it will take you.

A traumatic birth may also bring difficulty into your Mother phase. Pain, fear, and the feeling of being invisible and unheard can wreak havoc and destruction. We are all birthing our earthly babies in different ways. Some births are beautiful and ecstatic. Some go smoothly and rather fast. Some are lengthy but bearable and some bring forth a terrible trauma—all are equally important, and all should be debriefed. If you are a mother and have never done that before, think now, how was your birthing experience? Did you feel heard and respected? Were your hopes and preferences met? Did you feel fulfilled and happy afterwards, or more like a failure? Did you discuss your birth afterwards, or are you still frightening pregnant ladies with the horror stories from your delivery room? How do you feel about birth in general and how do you feel about being a mother? And then look back to your cycle, especially the Mother phase. How do you feel in this phase now? Do you struggle? What feelings, emotions, and memories are brought up from your unconscious? You can still work on that. You can reclaim your birth and grow in strength and feminine power. Are you ready?

During your Mother phase, you will find yourself deeply rooted in Mother Earth. You will become grounded and more insightful. You may choose to wear clothes that are more earthy in style and colour.

The Mother phase holds great depth and that may come forth through your clothing; through the way you move and interact with the world. With your deepening sexuality and inner strength and confidence you may find yourself more attractive to men. The best expression of the Mother phase is the body itself. If you have the opportunity to walk naked, please try it and feel the freedom it brings. Bare your breasts to the sun and breeze, allow the expression and openness to bring you closer to nature and the creative energies of life fully flow through you.

But if you suppress the free flow of your cycle, you may find the Mother phase totally different. You won't feel grounded, you will feel heavy, and the flow of creativity will be slow and sluggish or will stop altogether and you will feel stuck. You won't find freedom expressed through your body, but embarrassment and shame. Your body once again will become a tool of sin, and your horizon will combust. Your sexuality will become a burden and humiliation, and the needs of your body will mortify you. If those feelings will surface, be with them, acknowledge them as equally important and observe where they are coming from. That's the place that needs healing and you can call on your inner-mother or wait for the Wise Woman phase to help you out. Do not neglect or reject anything that comes up. It is all valid and important. It will all lead you to healing and wholeness.

The Mother phase offers an opportunity for great joy and happiness. You can find them in the giving of yourself, your abilities, love, attention, and help to others. The Mother phase allows you the ability to take on responsibility for yourself and others, to care for them and love them, offering guidance and compassion. You can use your strength and wisdom to offer help and advice but notice if you are staying in the domain of a Good Mother. A Terrible Mother will force her own views. She won't be fuelled by compassion, but by her own agenda and often fear and shame. A Terrible Mother will make you give off too much of yourself. She will suck your strength and confidence leaving you dry and exhausted.

The Mother phase can be a time to visit your own mother. To see her as the source of your life but at the same time to realise that although you are her child, you are also her equal as a woman—with your own strength, power, and wisdom, and just like she did before you—you are trying to do the best you can. With your mother, you can see the spiral of life circling back through generations and into the past, to your ancestors. But you can also see it reaching out into the future and you are both a vital part of this process. Remember, when your grandmother was pregnant with your mother, you were already within her; and when your mother was pregnant with you, the ovum that will become your child, was already within you as well. Generations within generations— a sacred spiral of life. And if you have young children, try to spend more time with them during this phase—a special time. You are influencing the world around you with your cycle—this is the most potent time for teaching, bonding, and creating sacred and special rituals that may change and deepen their lives and help them, if they are daughters, in their understanding and appreciating their own cycles.

The Mother phase can be very spiritual. It can bring a feeling of harmony with nature, with other people and with the divine. Allow yourself this time with nature. Sit quietly with Mother Earth and become part of her. Awareness of nature is very important, especially if you live in the city. Experience nature around you at night. Experience the sensations and emotions that come with the darkness, connect to the moon, to the stars. Although the summer of ovulation is the time of the full moon, your Mother phase can come at any moon phase. Notice what is happening in the sky and how does it affect you. How does the moon influence your cycle, your different phases? How do you connect with her? And if you haven't thought about it yet, this is a perfect moment to start. The sexuality of this phase brings a very strong creative drive. Notice how the moon phases influence your creativity and sexuality. How does the moon hold you?

The totem animal of our summer place in the cycle is the snake. The snake is a lunar animal too. She is the lunar animal because she also changes by shedding her skin. We can learn from the snake how to shed our skin whole, how to leave the past behind, how to die and be re-born again—this is a powerful wisdom. This is wisdom feared by many, and most of all feared by the patriarchy. This is why it was the snake in the Garden of Eden that promised this wisdom to a woman. Patriarchy wants us to believe that it was the birth of the first and greatest sin. But was it? Notice what was the first thing Adam and Eve saw after eating the forbidden fruit. They noticed their nakedness and felt shame for the first time. The rabbis said that menstruation was the result of Eve's relations with the serpent in the Garden of Eden, and in many cultures, women were seduced by them into their blood and sexual awakening. In many cultures snakes and the moon are identified. But the Divine Feminine doesn't perceive nakedness as shameful. It's natural to her.

So is her sexuality, sensuality, and body. This is where she takes information from and how she sits in the universe. And the snake is not the devil. This is the guide to the fullness of this wisdom. She is our mirror. She is the envoy of Nature, her emissary. And Mother can hear and understand this message. So together with the snake coiled around the moon, travelling the sky, and shedding her skin, so is the woman, changing constantly, shedding phase after phase, dying, and being born anew. She is the witch, as the witchcraft was bestowed by the moon. She is a shapeshifter. A woman is an embodied goddess.

The light and openness of the Mother phase can begin the earthing of the creative energy from the dark womb of the Crone. This light radiates forward into the world, cradling all life. The bright moon is the embodied dark moon, and creation is the manifestation of the divine. Ovulation brings the feeling of belonging to creation. It brings the joy of living, of being, brings richness and fertility. Ovulation with Lover and Mother archetypes opens itself to the direction of the South. And the South is the direction of creativity, sexuality, inspiration, and passion. South is revelation and fire. Fire is filled with the spirit, with the breath of life, with possibility. But fire, if untamed, can also be deadly. In each cycle, we can bathe ourselves in the noon of the summer day, in warmth and bliss. And it all depends on us whether we come home to ourselves with a beautiful and healthy glow or burn to dust.

CHAPTER 9

Dancing with goddesses: from Lover to Mother

Aphrodite

Aphrodite is the Greek goddess of passion, beauty, love, sensuality, and sensual relations with Earth. She was associated with the planet Venus. Aphrodite's name means 'foam born', and legend says that she sprang from her father Uranus's castrated genitals, which were cast into the ocean. Called Venus by the Romans, she was the icon of feminine beauty. She was widely worshipped as the goddess of the sea. The less common fact is that she was also honoured as the goddess of war at Sparta, Thebes, and Cyprus. However, fertility and love were her main attributes. Many scholars believe that her worship came to Greece from the East and is connected to the ancient Middle Eastern goddesses Ishtar and Astarte. Aphrodite took divine and mortal lovers and was also the patron goddess of prostitutes. Aphrodite was almost always accompanied by Eros, the god of lust and sexual desire. Her main attendants were the three Charites—Aglaea 'Splendour', Euphrosyne 'Good Cheer', and Thalia 'Abundance'. Aphrodite was a capricious goddess. She generously rewarded those who honoured her, but also brutally punished those who disrespected her. Her sacred animals were dolphin, sparrow, dove, swan, hare, goose, bee, fish, and butterfly.

Her symbols are rose, seashell, pearl, mirror, lettuce, and narcissus. Her trees are myrrh, myrtle, apple, and pomegranate. Aphrodite represents unabashed female sexual energy. She helps women discover and feel comfortable with their bodies and sexuality. She helps people experience more passion in their relationships and to become more balanced in their inner male-female energy representations. She shines with radiant love and sensual pleasure allowing us to discover the possibility of transformation through love and sex. You may call upon her to aid your inner work with self-worth, self-beauty, body acceptance and your feminine stand within the world. She may aid you in regaining your inner strength, power, and beauty. She can be gentle, but she will also show you the truth of who you are and who you are able to become. Just look into her mirror and see for yourself.

Questions to journal with

– What does connecting to the Lover archetype mean for me?
– What does connecting to the Mother archetype mean for me?
– How does the Lover show itself in my life?
– How does the Mother show itself in my menstrual cycle?
– What do I wish to share and express?
– What support do I need to birth my visions?
– Which of my gifts are ready to be offered into the world?
– What does being in the world mean to me?
– What does sacred service to myself mean to me and how will it emerge in my life now?
– Which one of my mother's wounds is holding me back?
– How do I connect to sacred sexuality and what does it mean to me?
– Where was the moon on her journey when I was travelling through my Lover and Mother archetype?
– How does the moon mirror the way I feel?

Rediscovery of pleasure practice

If you are ready, Aphrodite will take you on a journey to discover or rediscover your pleasure. Through this practice, you can get to know yourself intimately and truly. You will also be able to understand that you are the sole pleasure giver to yourself. You do not need the other for that. You are all that you need. But also, if you allow yourself this time of discovery, you will be able to open yourself more easily to the other person when the time comes. During this practice, you can call upon the goddess, build an altar for her and invite her to be your witness. You can also submerge yourself in your own sensuality without divine intervention. Have a beautiful journey.

Create sacred space

In this practice, you are going to hold yourself in the highest regard and with the most respect. Make it beautiful for yourself. Light the candle, burn incense, and smudge your space to clear it of negativity and profane energy. Create a beautiful nest for yourself. It doesn't matter if it's a bed, sofa, or the floor—gather cushions and blankets, so you can be warm and comfortable. If your surroundings look nice, you will feel pretty good yourself. Take your time, you are not in any hurry. This is not a quick-fix masturbation. Orgasm is not the goal here. Pleasure is. So, darken the room and put on some nice music. Get naked or put on a nice floaty dress that won't constrict your movements and will be easy to lift or take off altogether later in your practice. Put on nice jewellery or scarves. Imagine how you would prepare your room and yourself to receive the lover of your dreams, and then give yourself exactly that. You are a lover of your dreams.

Welcome yourself to this sacred space. Be open to all the emotions and feelings that will come to the surface. You may already begin to feel emotional or tearful. Allow that to happen, do not stop the flow of energy. Let everything out. Let the energy flow freely through your body and energetic field. Make sure that you are always feeling safe. You can stop this practice at any moment. Even if creating the sacred space is enough, don't judge yourself. Flow with everything that comes up. Maybe next time you will venture further. Before each step ask yourself permission to carry on. Listen to the answer and respect it. Remember you can repeat this practice as many times as you wish, and you can stop at any part. Be kind and compassionate to yourself. Make sure that you have tissues, water, and maybe a nice snack ready. When you get into your nest, you may not want to leave it for some time. Is your sacred space set? Are you ready?

Show yourself love

Look down at your beautiful body. Your body carried you throughout your life to this point, through ups and downs, health and illness. Look at yourself truly, at the goddess that you are. Worship yourself, you are worthy of worship. Take a mirror and look at your beautiful *Yoni*. Say a prayer of gratitude to your *Yoni*. Describe what is beautiful about her and what you are grateful for. This is the moment in which you have an opportunity to change the emotional imprint associated with your body from one of shame and judgement to one of celebration and self-love. Take your time. This moment is very important. Your beautiful vulva is an entrance, a gateway to your sacred temple, to the portal of your womb. Isn't she amazing? Isn't she beautiful? Yes, she is. Take your time. See yourself truly in your own beauty.

Set the intention

Intention setting is an important part of each sacred practice. Think for a moment why are you here? What would you like to change or achieve through this practice? Intentions can be very simple or deeply spiritual, they are all equally important. What is your intention?

– Would you like to discover more about your sacred sexuality?
– Would you like to connect more with your goddess nature?
– Would you like to open yourself to new states of spiritual realisation?
– Would you like to discover pleasure or maybe greater pleasure?
– Would you like to explore and accept your sexuality?
– Would you like to explore and accept your *Yoni*?
– Would you like to heal past pain?
– Would you like to spend more time with yourself?

What is it that you need right at this moment? When setting your intention don't forget to state through I, for example, I would like to connect to my goddess nature. The intention of this practice is to connect to my goddess nature. If you wish so, repeat your intention three times.

Create the feeling and experience of total acceptance for yourself

Remember, magic is in the slowness. During your practice don't rush yourself. Don't pressure yourself, don't judge, or criticise yourself in any way.

Put one hand over your heart and one over your womb. Hold yourself in this beautiful heart-to-womb connection. Breathe deeply. Imagine your breath travelling between your heart space and your womb space. Allow it to flow, gently and easily. When you are ready, breathe down into your womb space and move the hand from your heart down to your vulva. Keep the other hand over your womb space. Now breathe deeply in and out and allow the energy of your breath to travel between your womb space and your vulva. Allow the breath to reach your vulva, allow your vulva to open underneath this breath. Allow yourself to feel peace and full acceptance. If any judgement creeps in, that's okay. Gently and with compassion realise the judgement and remember your intention. You are allowing yourself to go deeper and to open new and deeper states of full acceptance. It's a journey and you are not in a hurry. You may feel that you have touched your edge now, and it's ok to stop the practice if that is your wish. Just hold yourself, allowing any emotions that arise to flow through you. Look at yourself with love and kindness. Accept where you are today. But if you are ready, I invite you to dive deeper.

Full body self-massage

Start at the place you feel most comfortable with. It could be your hand, or shoulder, stomach, or thigh. Gently stroke your body. Touch yourself as you've always longed to be touched. Don't think of this practice as a lover substitute. Instead, touch yourself as if you are the most amazing, precious, and loved person in the entire world. You are your own sacred beloved. Embody it fully. Stroke yourself all over your body. Slowly, gently—discover different types of pressure and touch. What gives you pleasure? Follow the song of your pleasure. Rub your arms, your belly, and thighs, and massage your breasts. Touch yourself wherever you desire to be touched. How about your face, your neck, ears, hair, fingers? Let go and become the touch. Become the feeling of being touched. While you are stroking your body try to take deeper and deeper breaths. This is meditative practice and touch is your meditation. This is an embodied touch. Relax further with each breath. Pay attention to the sensations in your body. Notice them and let them go, don't hold on to anything. Allow it to be in constant flow.

Stroke your inner thighs

Start to stroke your inner thighs. Slowly and gently. If that is enough for you, leave it at that, and explore your inner thighs. If you would like to venture further, start on your inner thighs, then stroke over your hips, your belly and back down over your vulva and into the thighs. Repeat it gently and slowly. Change the direction of your movement, the speed. What is your body telling you to do? How does it feel? What feels the best? If you start feeling turned on, that's fine. If you are not turned on, that's fine as well. Explore your pleasure. Be gentle, compassionate, and full of love for yourself. You can stroke anywhere and in any way that feels good.

Tune into your bliss

Start to notice what feels super pleasurable. Do gentle strokes bring you more pleasure or maybe the firmer ones? Can you feel connected to yourself and your pleasure? Are you madly in love with yourself yet? If not, don't worry, take your time. It will come. This practice is a touch meditation. Meditating on pleasure, experiencing it with each inhale and each exhale. Breathe deeply. Seek what feels good without pushing yourself, without expectations. If your thoughts wander, that's okay. Notice that and bring them back to your body. In this practice you are not to fantasise or imagine erotic scenarios, you can do that another time and enjoy it fully too. In this practice, you are giving in to the pleasure, of feeling with your entire body and all the senses. That's it. Breathe deeply.

Clitoral play

If you are ready to explore more, run your fingers over your clitoris. How does it feel? Does she like gentler strokes or firmer ones? Touch her in a way that feels amazing to you. If you feel yourself wanting to orgasm, slow down, and focus back on your pleasure. Your pleasure is all that exists in this moment. Nothing else matters. No expectations, no end goal you need to reach. Just the present moment and you, your body, and your touch.

Inner exploration

Are you ready to dive deeper? Breathe deeply in and out. Start to explore the opening of your vagina with one or two fingers. Ask your Yoni—is it alright today to be explored in this way? Listen for the answer. If the answer is no, go back to your clitoral play and explore your body in this way. If the answer is yes—gently slide your fingers inside, delicately slipping and sliding. Touching the front and back wall, touching the sides. How far in would you like to go? What brings you pleasure? Breathe deeply, slide in and out, be present. You are making pleasure the object of your presence. Your body, your feelings, this meditation is your sexual exploration. If other feelings surface, be fully with them. The truth lies within, and within you is the portal to your personal power. As you explore your inner vagina and become more intimate with yourself, with all the sensations, you will go deeper into the experience and deeper into knowing yourself.

Breath

At any point when your pleasure is building, deepen your breath. We've been taught over centuries that we feel pleasure, that we can orgasm on contraction. We can because this is what we have learnt. But please try for a change to get to the top of your pleasure during expansion. Allow your body a contraction-free experience. Breathe directly into your pleasure. Breathe deeply. As you do this, drop more and more into the sensations, and use your breath to allow yourself to touch your divinity. By breathing in this way, you will enter an altered state of reality and you will be able to meet yourself on an entirely different level.

Surrender

Listen to your body. What does it want to do? Allow your hands to have a life of their own and your pleasure to be your guide. Touch yourself in the way you want to, go wild, and let yourself surrender fully into this moment and into your body. Now is the time to be free. It's the time of the ecstasy. Allow all the emotions out. If you feel like crying, cry. If you want to laugh, do it. If you want to slow down or stop, go for it. Surrender.

Orgasm

If you start to feel orgasmic, breathe into it. Relax your entire body and go for it. When you surrender in this way into pleasure, into your body, your entire consciousness opens and activates. You can reimprint the way you thought you should orgasm or live. You can heal the past, present and the future. You are fully open, and the energy is flowing right through you.

Thanksgiving

Hold your body. Your beautiful, amazing, gorgeous body. Hold yourself tightly. Now think and say out loud three things—three things you are grateful for with your body and for this experience. Say them out loud so you can hear them. Thank your body for being this incredible vessel, this beautiful temple.

Remember that your life is your journey. Sometimes you can fully explore and give in to pleasure, but sometimes very hard lessons and wounds will come to the surface. Sometimes you may feel blockages, or issues or you may realise there is so much to heal. Don't be discouraged. This is a beautiful path to healing, and you are walking it already. You are setting intentions and then using tools to be present for anything that comes up. Your body is your perfect tool. It's your friend and helper. So, whatever comes, thank yourself, your guides, your goddess, and trust that you are in alignment with your path, with your intuition and with your body. You are in alignment with your higher self.

Note on lube

I would highly recommend using lube with this practice. There are many available on the market, but for me the best one on the market at the moment is Yes, Water-based Personal Lubricant. It is UK-based, certified organic, hormone and glycerine free lubricant. I absolutely love it. If you are interested, you will find the link to her online store in the 'Useful links' section at the end of this book.

Freya

Freya is the Norse goddess of love and fertility; she hails from the family of deities known as Vanir, fertility gods. Her residence is a beautiful palace called Folkvang ('field of folk'), a place where love songs are always in the air. She was given this place by the gods of Asgard, who were so very charmed by her beauty and grace. She is considered to be a divine female of raw sensuality and vigorous passions, who is not shy about expressing herself. She was the most beautiful and beloved of all the goddesses, and while in Germany she was identified with Frigga, in Norway, Sweden, Denmark, and Iceland she was a goddess by herself.

Although the goddess of love, Freya was also hardened by her martial tastes. As a leader of Valkyrie, she often led them down to the battle-field choosing and claiming one half of the heroes slain. This is why she was often represented in her corselet, helmet, shield, and spear in a chariot pulled by two mighty cats. Freya would transport the chosen slain to Folkvang, where they would feast and have a wonderful time. She would also welcome there all pure maidens and faithful wives, so they could enjoy the company of their lovers and husbands after death. Freya was believed to favour lovers' prayers and she was often invoked by them in love songs.

Sometimes she was considered as personification of Earth. As a god-dess of beauty, she adorned herself with beautiful garments and jew-els. She was given the most wonderful necklace—Brisingamen—by the dwarves, after promising to grant them her favour. As she was also considered the goddess of fruitfulness, she was sometimes represented riding together with her brother Frey in a chariot drawn by the golden-bristled boar, scattering fruit and flowers for mankind. But her favourite chariot was the one drawn by cats, her favourite animals, the emblems of sensuality and fertility. Frey and Freya were held in such a high honour throughout the North that their names, in modified forms, are still used for 'master' and 'mistress', and one day of the week is called Freya's day or Friday by English-speaking nations to this day. Freya was invoked for success in love, prosperity, and increase, but also for aid and protec-tion. Her sacred animals were swallows, cuckoos, cats, boar, falcons, ladybirds, rabbits, and horses. Her sacred tree was a sweet-smelling linden tree, almond and cypress. Her sacred plants were arnica, daisy, clover, hemp, mugwort, opium poppy, primrose, rose, and strawberry.

Unafraid of her sexual power, Freya teaches us to appreciate our attractiveness, and to enjoy ourselves. You can call upon her to aid you with releasing inhibitions. You can also work with her to magnetise love and passion through the natural expression of your feminine energy. She is also a goddess of sacred polarity, and as such she walks between light and dark, birth and death, love and war. She is a beautiful example of the depths of a goddess's divinity and in this way also mirrors the divinity of each woman. She will aid you in your deeper connection to your sensuality and sexuality. She will also aid you in creating self-care and self-love rituals to discover your beauty and potential. She can teach you to be yourself unapologetically and to face the world.

Temple of beauty practice

When Freya wears her precious magical necklace, her allure intensifies and people as well as gods fall under her spell. You can begin this practice by buying yourself a new Freya necklace. Or maybe you already have one. One that was too extravagant or too much to wear so far. When you choose your necklace, bless it with your intention and imagine that it has magical powers to draw in your desires. What is your intention? Would you like a spicy love life? Would you like to deepen your feminine power? Would you like to connect to your feminine energy? Or maybe you would like to find beauty in yourself and the surrounding world? Whatever your intention is pull it all into your necklace.

When you finish, take all your clothes off and dress yourself solely in your neckless. How does it feel? Stand in front of the mirror. Look at yourself with love and compassion. Look at yourself truly, like you've never looked before. What can you see? Can you see only the projections of others or can you notice your beauty as well? It may not be easy, standing like that in your vulnerability. But please don't cover yourself up. Look at your naked body. It has been serving you for so long. Notice yourself, maybe for the first time. If it's too much you can finish the practice at any time without judgement and maybe get back to it tomorrow. But if you can then please look fully, with love and longing. Tell yourself what you can see. But say only the nice things. You have others to point to all the rest. What can you see? I can see the goddess that you are. Dressed in your power amulet, can you feel it? Breathe deeply and look. Touch your body and feel its response. Embrace yourself, hold yourself, and give yourself time. We are beautiful just the way we are. We are the beauty canon creators, and I am my beauty canon.

When I look into the mirror like that, I can see that I am beautiful just the way I am, and my body is a witness and a map of my past adventures and hardships. It's a map of who I have become, and who I grew to be, and I am proud of it. Each of my scars tells the story of the battles I fought—a battle with a broken spine, a battle with cancer, and the one where my body opened wide so the new life could come through. Why should I be embarrassed by them? Why should they be hidden? Each of these battles shaped the woman I am today. Each holds its own truth, beauty, and life lesson. Let me tell you what I can see now when I lovingly look into the mirror. My body holds in itself the magic of metamorphosis. It changes, but so do I. I'm growing as a person and my body is different than 20 years ago—bigger, softer, and cuddlier. I metamorphosed from an innocent girl into a conscious woman. From budding breasts of youth to mature ones filled with life-giving sustenance of motherhood and sexual pleasure. From hips straight in girlish innocence to ones curved with wisdom, strength, and flexibility of childbearing. To hips wide enough to find support for my own physical and emotional needs, and wide enough to let a child shelter safely behind. From legs created for running and chasing in childhood to those that take me places, propel me, and ones becoming the band for encircling a lover.

My body protects, supports, and contains. But my body is also a repository of memory. Everything that happens to me, the good, the bad, the beautiful, and the ugly, imprints itself in my soft tissues and in my bones. It comes out when touched, when pressure is implemented and held—and that brings me healing and aids in processing my past. It also provides supreme psychic and emotional nourishment. The held-in memories are important. They are necessary and they can lead not only to healing and peace but also to growth and the ability to move on. My body gives me grounding, weight and is filled with feelings. It can be touched, caressed, and loved, but it can also be hurt and abused. My body teaches me who I am and shows me my physical place in the world. My body does all that and so much more. Why shouldn't I look at it with gratitude? Why should I compare it to anything else? Our bodies are beautiful, and, in their beauty, they cannot be too much of this or not enough of that. They are what they are.

So, please look again in your mirror. What can you see?

Walk around your home naked. Allow your necklace to catch the sun's or moon's rays. How does it feel? If you feel daring, go into your garden. Walk naked around the trees and plants. Allow the sun or moon rays to caress your body. Can you feel the freedom? Free yourself from judgements and expectations. If you don't have a garden put on the floating dress and don't wear anything underneath. Go out like that. Find a place in nature where you will be able to sit on the ground. Your *Yoni* on Mother Earth. How does it feel? Breathe deeply. Find your inner goddess. Connect to your inner love and beauty and the outer ones will follow suit.

You can wear your necklace whenever you need additional support, strength, or love.

Gaia

Also spelt Gaea—Grecian Primordial Being, Creatrix of Life, Earth. A cosmic, procreative womb that was believed to have emerged out of the primaeval void called Chaos. She existed before all other life. A supreme power who created everything—the entire universe, all the deities, plants, animals, and humans. She is called an 'all-producing and all-nourishing' goddess, The Mother. She may have been an earlier Phoenician goddess adopted by Greeks as their own. She had many children, some by herself, some by merging with a male deity. She was the mother of the first race—the Titans. Although she was powerful unto herself, she didn't choose a solitary existence. From her womb, she formed the Sea, which she called Pontus, and the Sky, which she called Uranus. The Sky lay upon the Earth seeding her fertile womb. The Sea filled her womb with all primordial sea gods. Through her union with Sea and Sky, Aether and Hemera came to be. These two children later became known as Night and Day. In artwork, she is represented in different forms. One of the oldest vase paintings from Athens depicts her as an older woman and matronly figure, with half of her body still in the ground. There are also paintings representing her as a younger and very beautiful woman. The most common epithet associated with her is Anesidora 'giver of gifts'. Her cult was tightly woven with that of Demeter, and both goddesses were worshipped equally. Gaia was the original oracle and there is a legend saying that she was the creator of Delphi. As Great Mother, she was viewed as the ultimate ideal of femininity and fertility. Mother Earth disappeared from popular mythos until James Lovelock brought her back. He introduced the Gaia hypothesis. This theory claims that both inorganic compounds and living organisms on the planet must work together.

Gaia is teaching us that everything on Earth is connected and that in reality we are all one living, breathing organism. She is teaching us respect and owe to all of life and creation. Call Gaia if you need help with grounding, feeling present in your own life, and embodying your life and needs. You can ask her for help in any process of creation. As a primordial womb, she will help you to connect to your own womb and work with your cycle. She is also our Great Mother. She will help you feel loved and accepted when your mother's wound is becoming too strong to bear. She will also accept you when you decide to be born Earthwise, consciously and with purpose. By trusting her, you are trusting in the power of the womb, femininity, and truth. By following her you can become the creatrix of your own life. As creatrix, the Earth is trying to dream creation forward and now she operates through us, through people alive currently. This is why through connecting with the Mother, diving deeply into her womb we are re-discovering the power of our own wombs, the creative gifts lying within. And if we have enough courage to descend, we will be rewarded with gifts and ideas, visions and courage, everything that is needed to forge and to keep the creation going.

The spiral walk

I would highly recommend doing this practice outside, in nature, feeling the earth underneath your feet. But if for any reason you cannot go out right now, you can also do it at home. If in nature, please find sticks, twigs, leaves, flowers, stones, or yarn. When at home, you can use whatever you can think of. Using all your gathered materials, please build a spiral on the ground that is large enough to walk through with at least three turns and the space in the middle to sit down. If you are working at home and cannot sit on the ground, you can place a chair in the middle of your spiral. If your room is not big enough, build an outline of the spiral and you can walk it in your visualisation/imagination. The intention is the most important thing in this practice, not the perfect spiral.

The shape of the spiral is present everywhere in nature. Its shape, one of a coiled serpent, has been used since ancient times as a tool for growth and transformation. A spiral guides us when we enter deeply within our consciousness and unknown, it extends far out into the heavens, and deep down within the fertile darkness of Mother Earth. The direction you are going to travel in is up to you.

Build your spiral. Look at it for a moment and then enter it slowly. Walk your spiral with the intention of going within, whatever it means to you at this moment in time. Walk it slowly and mindfully. Once you reach the centre sit down and place one hand on your womb and the other on the earth. Breathe deeply and feel your body relaxing. Your breath is becoming deeper and longer. If it feels comfortable to you, close your eyes. Feel Gaia underneath you. Feel her truly. Feel yourself supported and held. If you are ready offer to the Great Mother Earth all feelings and situations that you no longer want in your life, that no longer serve you. Feel them flowing from your womb into the womb of the Mother. Give yourself as much time as you need. When you feel complete, imagine that from your womb mighty roots are growing out and anchoring you in Mother Earth. Feel those roots growing down and down, through the fertile soil into the core of our beautiful planet. Through these roots, you are going to breathe with Gaia.

On the in-breath bring up from within the core all the nutrients and grounding that you need. On the out-breath, give back your love and gratitude. Feel them flowing back into Mother Earth and nurturing her in exchange. Breathe like that with Gaia for a while. When you feel complete, say a prayer of gratitude, and bring the roots back up into your womb. Feel them dissolving back into your own womb. When you can feel yourself fully back in your body open your eyes. Stand up and walk the spiral in the opposite direction. Walk back to the way you entered. As you do, feel recharged and rejuvenated, feel grounded, and present. Feel ready for your new journey. When you finish walking your spiral, thank Mother Earth, your guides, the spiral medicine. If you build your spiral from natural material, you may leave it as an offering to nature. Turn around and walk away. You are leaving the old behind, there is no reason to look back. If you created your spiral at home, pick up the items, open the window and leave the room for a moment without looking back. Feel refreshed and recharged. Feel connected to the web of life and your Great Mother.

PART 4

ENCHANTRESS—THE POWER OF THE SHAPESHIFTER

CHAPTER 10

Placenta—the gift of life

The placenta is an organ that develops in the uterus during pregnancy. It provides oxygen and nutrients for the growing baby and removes waste products from the baby's blood. The placenta attaches to the wall of the uterus and connects to the baby by the umbilical cord. What's amazing about the placenta is that it is a temporary organ, created for the needs of maintaining the pregnancy, and that it produces hormones that regulate both mother and the baby. History teaches us that the placenta first evolved in mammals about 150 to 200 million years ago. The protein syncytin, found in the outer barrier of the placenta between the mother and the baby, has a certain RNA signature in its genome that has led to the hypothesis that it originated from an ancient retrovirus—a virus that helped with the transition from egg-laying to life-birth. This virus also helped primates to fight off other viruses by preventing them from entering cells ('Ancient Virus May Be Protecting the Human Placenta', *Science*, 27 October 2022).

There are new studies that show this virus might have been a great help in developing the placenta in the way it can protect embryos from viral infections and that the evolution of the placenta may not have been possible without it. There is so much we don't yet know about the placenta. But the research is ongoing and new findings emerge each day.

The placenta has an important place in cancer studies. Research by Dr Erin Macaulay shows that 'the placenta, the wonder of human reproduction, is now providing insight into the invasive nature of cancer' (this research is being carried out in the Department of Pathology at the Dunedin School of Medicine, University of Otago). Her research focuses on genes that regulate the growth and development of the human placenta. She says that she was stuck by the similarities between the normal growth of the placenta and the abnormal growth of cancer, as the placenta starts to develop at the time of conception and rapidly invades the wall of the uterus. The difference is that after birth placenta breaks away and the uterus returns to normal. So maybe in this comparison there are the answers to the way how we can persuade the cancer cells to break away and leave our bodies. Just like I told you before, all the answers to the questions of the universe are held within a woman's body.

But the placenta is not only an organ. Its function for the growing baby is so much more than physical sustenance. The placenta is the protective pouch that forms around each and every one of us and takes care of us during our time in gestation in our mother's wombs. We are held by the placenta and that holding brings us peace and the feeling of safety. This is the feeling that we are trying to come back to repeatedly in our adult lives. This feeling of being held in safety, of being surrounded with protection and love. Everything is muffled down in the womb; everything is as it should be. In many cultures placenta is believed to be the baby's 'tween energy'. It is believed that the placenta has a consciousness that bonds with the baby, nurtures and takes care of the baby before he/she is born. This consciousness is bonded tightly with the baby and is our first teacher. When the umbilical cord is severed prematurely this can be an extremely traumatic experience, as the placenta is the baby's connection to feeling safe and nurtured. If it is severed too quickly, this can create a shock in the body and an energetic disconnection to our Great Mother—The Earth. Have you ever felt that you don't belong? That you don't belong to your family, to the country you are living in, to this planet, to your own body? Have you ever felt that this life doesn't belong to you, and you don't belong to this life? If yes, believe me, you are not alone in this feeling. The severing of our umbilical cord before we are ready to be born creates a trauma that we are facing for the rest of our lives. How often do we feel we don't belong? How often do we feel worthless? How often do we feel that we don't really exist?

We feel this way because we weren't allowed to be born consciously. We weren't allowed the time to transition from within our mothers and the safe embrace of the placenta into the without of the world and the embrace of our own bodies. We weren't allowed the time to make this transition consciously and on our own terms. Working as a doula blessed me with being present at many births. I am the witness to rushing and the trauma it brings. But I have also witnessed peace and the gift of time. I always wondered what different life those babies would have. To help with this transition as parents we can opt for delayed cord clamping and cutting. After birth, the cord is left attached to the baby until it stops pulsating and all the blood from the placenta is back with the baby once more. Then it is cut. Another option could be the Lotus birth. Lotus birth was quite common within Asian and African cultures. It was introduced to the US in 1974 and spread from there all over the world. In a Lotus birth, the placenta is left attached to the baby.

It is preserved with salt and herbs and carried in a pouch or bag with the baby. When the mother holds the baby, the bag is always with them. The child decides themselves when they are ready to let go and be born earthside. When the baby is ready to let go of this form of nourishment and safety, the umbilical cord simply falls off. The placenta is then buried in a sacred place on Earth to support the baby in having a strong and rooted connection to Mother Earth. So, even though the physical connection to the mother is there no longer, the energetic connection to Mother Earth is always with us. But one doesn't have to be the child of Lotus birth to be born consciously. In all energy work intention is what matters most. Even if we won't opt for delayed cord cutting for our baby, or the cord has been cut straight after delivery for any reason, the part of the placenta is still attached to it. This part can be treated as an energetic connection to the mother. If you hold your baby putting your hand over it, you can say out loud: 'We are still connected energetically to one another. We are not in a hurry. Stay connected in this way for as long as you need to and when you are ready, simply let go'. You can spend some time daily putting your hand over the clamp and talking to your baby. When they are ready the remaining cord will fall off and the belly button will form. We can then pick up the detached part and bury it in Mother Earth with the intention of creating an energetic cord connection between our babies and the Great Mother. This connection is extremely important and may help them to feel that they belong—to this planet, to this body, to this life.

But what about us? When I was born nobody thought twice of the importance of placenta and conscious birthing. My mother didn't have a choice, she was told not to worry her pretty head about anything, and the doctors knew what they were doing. Generations of children came to this world in this way. But nothing is lost—remember, intention is all that matters. We can go back in time and choose to be born consciously and take full responsibility for our own lives from now on. Because the feeling of not belonging, and feeling of not being worthy puts us in the position of the victim. Victims have things done to them; they have no choice. I don't want to be a victim anymore. Do you? I want to take full responsibility for my actions and thoughts. I want to create my own reality, and dream my life into being. Dream my own dream. Not somebody else's, my own—conscious, grounded, and present life. I am the creatrix and I have that power within me. And so do you.

I would like to invite you to do a beautiful ceremony for yourself. Ceremony that will help you to fully arrive on this planet and in your life. Ceremony that will allow you to take full responsibility for yourself, for your body, and your energetic field. Ceremony that will allow you to be born consciously earthside. And it doesn't matter that your birth may have happened 20, 30, 40, 50, 60, or more years ago. This one will herald your conscious choice of being born here and now, in this time and in this body, and will commence the life of the new you. During this ceremony, you will give birth to yourself and connect consciously with our Great Mother. After that everything becomes possible. First, we'll do conscious birth meditation together, and then I will invite you to perform a placenta burial ritual.

Conscious birth meditation

Find a comfortable position. You may sit or lie down. It is entirely up to you. How do you feel today? What is comfortable right now? Breathe easily and gently—in through your nose and out through your nose or mouth—you choose. How would you like to breathe today? Notice the cold air coming in through your nose, the air is warming up inside of your body and then the warm air is coming out of your mouth (or nose). Breathe like that for a moment, in and out, gently, naturally. Notice that with each breath your breathing is becoming slower and deeper, and that with each breath your body is becoming more and more relaxed. Each time you breathe in, allow yourself to open more space within you for the new to come, and each time you breathe out allow the old to leave your body. All that no longer serves you, allow it gently out on the out-breath. Without expectations, only with trust and curiosity.

Now I would like to invite you to begin the wave breath. On the in-breath take the energy and the breath from the bottom of your feet and allow it to travel up your body to the top of your head. On a gentle pause between in-breath and out-breath, allow this energy to linger at the top of your head, and then on the out-breath flow the energy and the breath down your body to your feet, then out of your feet and into Mother Earth. In and up, out and down. Breathe like that for a few in-breaths and out-breaths. Now, if you are ready, please place your hands on your womb. On the in-breath allow the breath and the energy to travel up to the top of your head, pause there for a second and on the out-breath allow it to slowly flow into your womb space. Slowly and gently, through your throat, through your heart—your mighty drum, right down into your womb space. Take as much time as you need. Breathe deeply in and out of your womb space. Allow the life-giving force of your breath to enter your womb. Breathe fully into your womb space.

You are in your womb space now. As your womb is a portal, you can travel through time and space. See the portal within your womb, submerge yourself fully in it and travel back in time and space to the moment when you yourself were in your mother's womb. Through the portal of your womb, through this beautiful connection, you are now in your mother's womb. Sense and feel the placenta surrounding you. This placenta is your support system, this is your twin. It holds space and energy for you within your mother's womb. It gives you breath, life, and sustenance. Allow yourself to feel this connection to your placenta right now. You are safe, you are being held, you are supported and loved. A living organism encased around you, supporting you with your every need. Breathe deeply. Your umbilical cord is attached to the placenta from your belly button. Feel yourself drawing in nutrients, energy, and life force through this cord and into your body. Feel your gratitude and your appreciation for and to your placenta now. Feel your deep connection to your placenta and what this connection means to you. What information is coming your way? What feelings, pictures, and sensations? Immerse yourself fully in all of them. Breathe deeply.

Now you feel ready to be born into this world. You can feel the downward pull, and everything is tightening around you. As you are leaving your mother's womb and travel through the tight birth canal focus on your umbilical cord that is still attached to your placenta. You can still feel the support that flows through your cord. You can still feel connection and love. As you come out into the world, you can still feel attached to your placenta. Feel strong contraction and great expansion filling in your body. You are born earthside. It's colder here, brighter, louder, but you are still connected to your tween energy, feel its pulse, feel the communication between both of you. You are being held in love, safety, and delight. You can feel yourself being held now in your mother's arms. She is cuddling you into her breast. Your umbilical cord is still attached to your placenta, to your tween energy source. Feel how important this connection is. The placenta is your safety and comfort, helping you to feel nourished and secure as you get accustomed to the new world, as you begin to breathe by yourself with the outside air. Allow yourself to trust in this process. You feel good, you can feel the touch of your mother's hands on your body, warmth on your skin. You can smell her milk. You are ready to disconnect from your mother, you are ready to disconnect from your placenta and become your own person. You can breathe for yourself, you can eat for yourself, and you are held in safety and love.

Trust the process, and you will feel your cord detaching from your placenta when you are ready. Stay in this place, feeling that trust and safety of not being rushed or forced. This is your choice, and you are making it now. When you are ready feel your umbilical cord naturally detaching itself, giving you your independence. You can feel the outside world and you have new ways of being nurtured, nourished, and sustained. Allow this process and transition to be smooth, on your own terms, in your own time. You are born. You let go. You are conscious, brave, and independent. You know that your needs are going to be met by your mother and by your inner-mother, who always lives within you. Allow this transition to be delicate and loving. Breathe deeply.

Now through the portal come back to your own womb. Your beautiful womb in your own body, in this time and this space now. You are back to your adulthood, your maturity, your power. You are back in your womb now. Breathe deeply into your womb. From the depth of your womb feel, sense, or see a beautiful cord extending downward and like a mighty root sinking into the earth. Allow this root to travel deep within the belly of our Great Mother. Allow it to travel as deep as feels right for you. Through this root, you are now connected to

Mother Earth. You can draw nutrients, grounding, and sustenance in time of need. You can give and take in beautiful communication and communion with the Earth. On each in-breath feel the energy and sustenance flow from Mother Earth into your body. When you pause for a second between in-breath and out-breath, feel this energy becoming stronger. On the out-breath send your love and gratitude down into the depths of Mother Earth. In beautiful communion and communication. In and out. Together with our beloved planet. Breathe like that with the Earth for a moment.

When you feel complete, slowly retract the root from the depths of Mother Earth into your body and into your beautiful womb. Take as many breaths as you need to bring this cord back into yourself. Breathe deeply. Now you are back in your womb again. Gather all this beautiful energy we were working with today and on the in-breath move it to your heart space, on the out-breath move it back into your womb space. Move this beautiful energy into your heart space, so you can feel your truth. You are safe and you are loved. On the next in-breath move this beautiful energy to your throat and on the out-breath back into your womb again. Move this beautiful energy to your throat, so you can speak your truth. You are heard, you are present. Now on the next in-breath move the energy from your womb to the top of your head and on the out-breath move it back into your womb space. We are moving this energy to your higher self, so you can know and remember your truth. You are strong, powerful, and independent. Now on the next in-breath move this beautiful energy to the top of your head and on the out-breath allow it to flow all over your body. Envelop yourself like in a cocoon in this nourishing energy. You are present; you are supported; you are grounded. On the next out-breath let everything go. Feel yourself coming back into your body. Gently move your fingers and toes. Stretch your neck and when you are ready, but only when you are ready, open your eyes.

Welcome back. Welcome to your body and to your life. Welcome to your strength and power. Welcome home.

Placenta burying ritual

Like with all rituals, intention is the most important part. Your intention for this ritual is to reconnect to all aspects of yourself and to reconnect to the grid of Mother Earth.

I would like to invite you to go for a conscious walk with the intention of finding in nature a representation of your placenta. Before you set off, hold this intention in your mind and then go for a beautiful walk in nature. While walking notice everything around you and if something will catch your attention approach it gently and quietly and ask if it would like to be a representation of your placenta. It could be anything—a rock, stone, stick, leaf. Listen for the answer. If the answer is no, say thank you and move forward with the walk. If the answer is yes, gently pick this object up, leaving a little gift behind. Your gift could be a prayer, or a bead, it could also be a piece of you—your hair or saliva. When you finish your walk thank the spirit of that place for help and beauty you have witnessed.

Now, when you have your placenta representation, you are ready for your ritual. Find a place in nature that is special for you, calls you, or a place you find beautiful and sacred. It can be your back garden as well. Choose a day that feels right for you, has any significance, or maybe even your birthday. Also, you can be guided by the phases of the moon. Which phase is calling you the most? Think about it. Also, choose the time that feels right. Remember, this is your ritual, you are in charge. To prepare your object, wait for your moon-time and decorate it with your menstrual blood. If you don't bleed anymore, you can use your ordinary blood if you wish so, your saliva or hair.

Go to your special place. Ask for permission. If the answer is no, you will have to find another one. If the answer is yes, dig a little hole in the soil. Stand above it and hold your placenta representation to your heart. Say out loud:

> I choose the conscious birth. I can feel you Mother underneath my feet. I can feel your energy, your grounding powers. I'm breathing with you and through you. I release all vows, oaths and agreements that have disconnected me from the creation grids of Mother Earth.

Place your placenta representation in the hole and say: 'I choose life. I am safe. I belong'.

Bury your placenta representation. Afterwards, place your hand on the soil and say:

> From this moment now I choose to align to the abundance of Mother Earth and her grids. I live in alignment with love, and truth

and I'm learning to walk the Beauty Way. I chose myself. I love myself and all of creation. So may it be and so it is.

Spend some time contemplating what has just happened. Send your gratitude to Mother Earth and to spirit, to gods and goddesses of your choosing. When you feel complete, return home.

CHAPTER 11

The shapeshifting Enchantress

The beauty of the Indian summer

Indian summer is my favourite season. In our Sun Medicine Wheel, it is a period of unseasonably warm, dry weather that occurs at the transition of summer to autumn. It is a time of ease, a breath of rest between the productivity of summer and the hectic preparation of autumn. The trees are beginning to let go and change their colours from green to beautiful golden, orange, reds, and browns, and the low sun shines through them in a majestic, almost magical way. Everything seems to be suspended in this dream-like reality. The warmth is still there but it is touched by the beginning of the change. The promise of the cold to come is in the air, tangible, and close. The forests, fields, and even cities are shrouded in this very special atmosphere. The world is set on fire with the beauty of colours and smells. The ability to let go of trees shows the depth of its beauty. Trees don't fight this change; they give in to it with natural trust and ease. And just before the end of this cycle's life, they stand straight in their beauty and power.

This is such a valuable lesson to us all. The heat of Indian summer is pleasant. Not the scorching blaze of the summer—it brings relief and respite. Life matured fully and now can be filled with its own magic.

Different to the fertility magic of the summertime. This magic promises darkness and the mysteries hidden within. The days are beginning to give space to the growing belly of the night, but within this change the energy is still dynamic and abundant. We are getting ready for the last harvest and beginning to prepare the larders for the autumn work. There is maturity in the air, but this maturity is different from the one we've experienced in the summer. This maturity is filled with knowing and power. This maturity touches the darkness and the death to come. This maturity allows us to shapeshift into new bodies and stands in the perfect balance between the darkness and the light. It is a powerful place to be.

Shapeshifter's powers and the gifts of post-ovulation

Enchantress energy is very powerful and for some women can be more dramatic than the Maiden phase. They both are times of this great dynamic energy that takes over our bodies and minds, but when the Maiden energy is directed outwards, The Enchantress energies are coming back inwardly. Physical strength and endurance are slowly decreasing, and you can become more agitated and restless. This restlessness can lead to frustration, anger, over-analysis, and guilt. You may direct it towards yourself or project it onto others. Some women can find themselves less able to deal with the problems and pressures that life puts on us every day. Some may find themselves truly overwhelmed. If that is what's happening, look back into your Mother phase. What happened there? What thoughts or decisions may need more processing or releasing? Are you worried that your conception plans may have been unsuccessful again? Is that where the guilt is rising from?

Give yourself a moment to take a deep breath in and out. You are past the ovulation, embrace the post-ovulatory magic. Breathe deeply, allow yourself some rest, and time out. Allow your body to begin to slow down. This is a special time. You are still filled with the buzz of ovulation, but your body is beginning to contract. Changing the flow, gathering back the troops you have sent out. Open your arms to receive them back. Open yourself to the change in this flow. This is where the magic delves. You can shape and twist it into form. You are the creatrix, the Great Shapeshifter. You can tap into any energy you want. For a little while you can become the Maiden if you wish so, or you can tap into Lover's strength and passion. You can revisit the Mother and if you are daring enough, you can channel the Crone/Sage energy and embody it fully. As Enchantress you can shapeshift into whatever form you want. The definition of enchantress is 'a woman who uses magic to put someone or something under a spell' (*Oxford Dictionary*). Claim this power now and put a spell on your own life. Embody it fully for growth, power, and healing. You can find your inner-witch, as during this phase you can become much more aware of your inner nature, and your spirituality. Your psychic abilities may increase, and your dreams may take on a magical theme. They can become the windows onto your soul.

During this phase, women can also find that their sexual energy is still very intense. You can feel incredibly sensual. This amount of sensuality can bring forth the memories of the Maiden-self, but unlike the Maiden when the sensuality is fun-loving and outwards directed, the sensuality of the Enchantress is on a more primal level. Enchantress can become self-assured in her sexual power, she can tease and seduce and can embody the original seductress whose powers men crave, find tempting and also utterly frightening. Enchantress sexuality can become quite aggressive, even vampiric (the succubus sucking out men's vital force and life), and often is directed towards self-gratification. You have mothered enough by that time in your cycle. Now it is time to take back in. But the secret is to hold everything in balance, as being just the succubus may leave you filled with guilt, and shame and ready to burst when the next phase will turn her face to look at you. The Enchantress is filled with eroticism. It is a different level than the one of the Lover. It's slightly darker and more mature. There is more daring and a lack of responsibility in this sexual energy. Energies cultivated and created during this phase can be tremendous and can be released as intense bursts of either creation or destruction. But remember from chaos come creation, so even the destructive outbursts can be turned into a creative flow.

Lover, Enchantress, and Sage intertwined

Enchantress has the power of the Lover deeply embedded in her body and psyche but at the same time she introduces and taps into the wisdom of the Crone/Sage—her own inner Wise Woman. All three combined create quite a strong magical trio. All are present within at the same time. This is why sometimes you may be feeling pulled in one or the other direction. But this is all okay. Just take your time, breathe, be curious. Explore yourself, your feelings, and your cycle. This is how you weave your magic. This is how you learn to shapeshift and connect to your power. Connect to the feeling of sensuality, eroticism, and your own witchiness and spin the magic from your womb. This is where your true wisdom resides. Stand in your power. Dress like an Enchantress would. Get lovely lingerie, jewellery, scarves. Flow with this energy from the inside out.

Towards the end of this phase, your breasts and belly may start to swell. Embrace them as they are and see them as the expressions of your erotic charm. Be erotic for yourself. Find pleasure and sensuality in everything you do. Do it for yourself, not for the other. Find Nirvana in your everyday activities, find it in now. Your sexual energy is very strong and mature. Your *Yoni* has been mapped fully. It is ripe with a post-ovulatory glow. There is no need to think about conception anymore. Your sex experiences can be free and adventurous. There is nothing that can stop you now. The exploration is for pleasure's sake only. Be in the moment with that feeling, and embrace it fully. Be the queen of your own private kingdom. Take your power in your own hands. If you cultivate this energy in such a fashion, there will be no space for frustration or restlessness, as all the energy will be directed into pleasure. And pleasure will fuel your creativity and will give you momentum to venture further. But listen to your body. Don't push too hard. Instead of pushing, try flowing, being, experiencing.

But eroticism is not the only strength of this phase. With Enchantress comes an increased need for awareness of your inner world, of this connection with your inner Wise Woman. What subject would satisfy your needs during this phase? Don't hold back—explore. Delve deeply into understanding your nature, dream, create rituals, play with herbs, and crystals, and find some kind of structure or an outlet for your needs, feelings and experiences. Enchantress is the best phase to learn about divination, so in the later phase you can fully embody your oracular power.

Towards the end of the Enchantress phase your awareness of the non-material world will become heightened. Your senses will sharpen, and that can propel your creativity in a physical but also more surreal way. You may become more aware of the supernatural side of the world, like walking in between the visible and the not visible one. Your dreams may become more vivid, and the messages may be coming in the waking state as well. Don't shut it out. Listen to everything your body, mind and soul are trying to tell you. Journal, remember, learn. This is a very important moment in your cycle, and it is preparing you for the descent. And even though you may not want to leave your higher ground—the descent is inevitable, and you cannot change that.

If you would interfere with this flowing force in any way, as the Enchantress phase progresses, you may become restless and emotional. Your power of concentration may decrease, and you may become increasingly illogical and sensitive. If that leads to a state of agitation, try relaxation techniques and meditation. This restlessness and frustration experiences may come from restrictions you put on your creative energies. You know this feeling of this is not good enough, why do I bother? If that comes up, try to explore where those thoughts are coming from. What blocks your creative process? Try not to be too intellectual about it.

The Enchantress phase is the phase of feelings and creative flow. It's not physical or intellectual, so don't get sidetracked with your mind playing tricks on you. Allow your body to be your guide. But at the same time acknowledge and listen to your intellect, so you can remain in a balanced state. If you find yourself unbalanced in those aspects, you may experience dramatic mood swings. By repressing your feeling body, and your creativity, by trying to deafen your intellectual capability, you will oscillate between physical and emotional highs and lows. This can lead to demanding behaviours, insecurity, hyperactivity, and depression. When you guide your creativity and give it an outlet; when you recognise the need to retreat and allow yourself to do so, you can discover that you have the ability to smooth your mood swings, befriend them and look at them in a more positive light. You will be able to discover the lessons they bring with them. And if the need for destruction enters the picture, channel it into positive destruction. Don't destroy other people by hurting them, don't hurt yourself. Instead, try to create something and then destroy it. Do a fire ceremony, and safely burn things in the fire pit. Punch the cushion, and stomp on the carton boxes until they flatten down like a pancake. Go to the forest and scream your frustration out. By letting it go, you will release yourself and allow the flow to take you further. Release the energy in the safest way.

The dark side of the Enchantress is a woman who is perceived as reproachful, argumentative, jealous, and admonishable. But we need to remember that this intolerance you may be feeling is born from frustration and anger with the world for not being able to meet your needs. The true core of things is of the utmost importance now, and society often will try to hide or lie its way around it. You may not have the patience for that any longer. The nearer you are to your Wise Woman phase, the more you will feel the need for expression of your inner truth. You will begin to speak your own mind and your inner truth. The secret is to remember the feelings of other people. And in the dark aspect of Enchantress, it is a hard thing to do. Trivial things that are usually easy to deal with can be blown out of proportion. The filters are coming down and you begin to say as it is, as you see it and feel it. It can be very seductive, to be able to express your own truth so easily, and you can forget that like all the other phases, this one is also only temporary. Again, only within the inner-balance you can find your solace. The balance between your truth and the pain it may cause. But please remember as well that underneath all that lies your need for personal change and growth. Don't take it away from yourself. Allow the space for that change, transition into it and allow it to take you to places yet unknown.

But the Enchantress phase is also a gateway to withdrawal—from the outside world, from society, group settings, into your own private cave. You may find that you are feeling less sociable, and that you are not so willing to offer others your time and energy. It's okay. If it is at all possible, find time for yourself. Far away from people and noise. Allow yourself some time to relax, rest and reconnect to your inner depths. Ask yourself a few questions. What changes do I have to make in my life at this moment? What can I use this energy for? Is there anything that needs to be born/created during this cycle, or am I done and ready for descent? Which of my needs are not being met and what can I do to meet them? Then try to find the answers, and if you can put them into practice. Use the pulsation of this energy to destroy/release the old and the unwanted from your life. Use it to break the ties that bound you to it. If the change may appear frightening during the other phases of your cycle, in the Enchantress phase it is very welcomed and necessary. Because this phase begins to weave your truthfulness, you are able to deeply look beyond the levels of illusion into what lies beneath and which parts of your life demand change. The Enchantress knows that everything is in constant movement, and that something must die, so the new can be born. The Enchantress bridges this knowledge from the inner world into the outer one.

The Enchantress begins the descent from the light into the darkness. She knows that she cannot ignore the changes she undergoes, and that she cannot repress the darkness of her nature. If she tried to attempt that, the bond between her body, mind, and her cycle would become broken and that would send her spiralling into oblivion. The trapped energy would focus on self-destruction and hate towards herself and the entire world. Enchantress is capable of finding her own true nature and she allows herself to act on it. As she becomes closer to her conscious and unconscious mind, she can discover that within the darkness lies the energies with the power of creation and destruction. She becomes the mistress of those energies, and she knows that she can weave them with compassion, love and nurturing, nourishing strength. She can combine creation and destruction within her body and allow that flow to take her into the place of her inner truth. She can tap into her shapeshifting powers to allow this energy to flow smoothly and to be directed into places of need. Through connection to her sexuality and sensuality, she can create the momentum and birth all that needs to be birthed before she will embrace the Wise Woman within. What an amazing power to stand in.

CHAPTER 12

Dancing with goddesses: the Enchantress

Hathor

In Ancient Egypt, Hathor was honoured and known as the Golden One—a goddess so powerful she could help with dilemmas ranging from love life to the lack of prosperity. As a goddess of fertility and plenty, she was believed to be mother to the pantheon of gods and goddesses. But she wasn't only the Mother Goddess, she was also a ruler of the underworld. She was the Giver of Life, but also the Destroyer of Life. Many identified Hathor with the Milky Way and honour her as a Mistress of Heaven. She was the goddess of many things: love, beauty, dancing, music, joy, sexuality, fertility, pleasure, and maternal care; she was also the protectress of women. In her role as goddess of beauty, she was the patron of cosmetics. Wearing cosmetics was often seen as a way to worship her, and mirrors and pallets of cosmetics were common offerings to this deity. She was the mother/consort of the sky god Horus, and also the daughter/consort to the sun god Ra. She was one of several goddesses who acted as the Eye of Ra—Ra's feminine counterpart, and in this form, she could connect to her vengeful aspect that protected Ra from all his enemies. Hathor was often represented as a cow or a woman wearing a headdress of cow horns and a sun disc.

This represented her maternal and celestial aspects. She was considered a Goddess Queen, ruler of fate and Queen Goddess of foreign lands and gods. Just as she crossed the boundary between Egypt and foreign lands, she could also pass through the boundary between the living and the land of the dead. This duality shows the true strength and might of Hathor as a deity. In her aspect of 'mother of mothers' she was considered a goddess of women, maturity, children, and work. Her mysterious energy connected with women and helped them in everyday life. Hathor was highly connected to turquoise gems, gold, and copper, and she was called the Mistress of Turquoise. Aside from her shape as a cow, she also took the form of a cat, lion, and goose. Her sacred tree was a sycamore tree, and its milky sap was regarded as the symbol of life.

Because of all her beautiful aspects, Hathor is the perfect goddess to call upon in the Enchantress phase. At the beginning of this phase, we are still filled with the maternal side that naturally cares for those in need and Hathor is teaching us that it must be balanced with receptivity, or the flow will be blocked. Receiving is the essence of feminine energy, yet we are often too busy with giving away to stop and consider it truly. We are taught that as women we must give, give, and give, yet the true aspect of femininity is the receiving and the flow. So often we feel bad about receiving gifts, or feel too ashamed to ask for help, and this type of attitude blocks our feminine flow. Receptivity is as natural as nurturing and giving energy and Hathor can help us to find this inner-balance. When we receive, we have more resources to give to others and to ourselves. Hathor can assist us in creating personal abundance. We can begin to notice everyday gifts and witness the bounty in nature and in our lives. But in her underworld aspect, Hathor is touching the wisdom of the Crone, of the Wise Woman who is waking up and ready to take over in the approaching new phase. In that way Hathor can perfectly balance us in the Enchantress phase and allow us to draw from all the other aspects of ourselves, she can help us to draw in everything that we need at this moment in time. Hathor can mother us in mothering ourselves, can help us to find inner-beauty, inner-wisdom, inner-balance, and connect to the wild women present in the world and in our bodies. Hathor can help us to call ourselves into now and draw from the Earth and from the heavens all the energy that we need to remain in a state of equilibrium and joy.

Inner-balance meditation

Create your sacred space

Lie or sit down comfortably. Breathe easily and gently—in through your nose and out through your nose or mouth—you choose. How would you like to breathe today? Notice the cold air coming in through your nose or mouth, the air is warming up inside of your body and then the warm air is coming out of your mouth (or nose). Breathe like that for a moment, in and out, gently, naturally. Notice that with each breath your breathing is becoming slower and deeper, and that with each breath your body is becoming more and more relaxed. Now I would like to invite you to begin the wave breath. On the in-breath take the energy and the breath from the bottom of your feet and allow it to travel up your body to the top of your head. On a gentle pause between in-breath and out-breath, allow this energy to linger at the top of your head, and then on the out-breath flow the energy and the breath down your body to your feet. In and up, out and down. Breathe like that for a few in-breaths and out-breaths. Become the wave of your breath. Hear each in-breath and out-breath. This is the ocean of your being, the ocean of your body. Embrace it fully. Now, if you are ready, please place your hands on your womb. On the in-breath allow the breath and the energy to travel up to the top of your head, pause there for a second and on the out-breath allow it to slowly flow into your womb space. Slowly and gently, through your throat, through your heart—your mighty drum, right down into your womb space. Take as much time as you need. Breathe deeply in and out of your womb space. Allow the life-giving force of your breath to enter your womb. Breathe fully into your womb space.

You are in your womb space now. How does she feel today? Does she have any messages, colours, or information for you? Maybe sounds, or smells? What is your womb showing you today? Stay with this feeling. Stay for a moment with your beautiful and wise power centre.

Now imagine that from the centre of your womb, a mighty root begins to grow. The root is growing down, out of your *Yoni* and into the soil of Mother Earth. Through the density of the soil, through rocks and other roots, your root is growing down and down. Right into the womb of Mother Earth. You can feel the moment it reaches the womb of Mother Earth, the energy and warmth, safety, and wisdom. Now on your in-breath breathe this energy from the womb of our Great Mother up your root and into your own womb, and on the out-breath breathe back into the womb of Mother Earth your love and gratitude. Beautiful womb-to-womb connection and exchange. Just your womb and the womb of Mother Earth. Stay in that communion for a moment.

Now, leaving the root deeply rooted within the womb of Mother Earth, bring your attention back to your womb. Take a deep breath in and on the out-breath allow another root (or a branch if that would be easier for you to visualise) to grow through your body upwards. Allow it to move through your heart, throat, head and out through your crown chakra. Allow this root/branch to stretch upward, through the sky, up into the universe, until it reaches the Cosmic Womb. You can feel the moment it reaches the Cosmic Womb, the energy, the tingling, the spaciousness, safety, and wisdom. Now on your in-breath breathe this energy from the Cosmic Womb into your womb, and on the out-breath breathe back into the Cosmic Womb your love and gratitude. Beautiful womb-to-womb connection and exchange. Just your womb and the Cosmic Womb. Stay in that communion for a moment.

Now, leaving the root/branch rooted deeply within the Cosmic Womb, bring your attention back into your womb. Take a deep breath in and on the out-breath flow down into the womb of Mother Earth. On the in-breath allow the energy from the womb of Mother Earth to flow into your body, through your womb and into the Cosmic Womb. On the out-breath allow the energy from the Cosmic Womb to flow down through your womb and into the womb of Mother Earth. Within your womb there is a knot, a centre, both energies meet there in perfect balance, and you breathe in infinity. In the shape of an eight (8), with the upper loop going through the Cosmic Womb; the lower loop rooting within Mother Earth's Womb and with the centre/knot within your womb. A beautiful exchange of energy between the womb of Mother Eart, your womb, and the Cosmic Womb. Between the wisdom of the Above and the wisdom of the Below. With you and your womb in the centre. In perfect balance. With all the wisdom gathered there, within your body. Within the perfect wisdom of the Great Within. Breathe deeply and allow this beautiful communion between the Great Above and the Great Below. The union that is happening within you. In this timeless place, with infinity. Breathe deeply and allow this exchange to happen. Witness it and embody it within your womb space. Stay in that communion for a moment.

Now allow yourself to come back into the knot of your womb. Release infinity. Slowly bring the root/branch from the Cosmic Womb back within the centre of your womb. Allow it to move slowly through the sky and back into your body through the crown chakra, then down through your head, throat, and heart until it reaches the centre of your womb. Now retrieve the root from the depth of the womb of Mother Earth. Do it slowly. Allow the root to slowly move upwards, through the fertile soil of Mother Earth, through your *Yoni* and back into to centre of your womb. Now within your womb, allow them both to dissolve into the walls of your womb, filling them with the wisdom and the memory of this exchange. How does your womb feel now? Breathe deeply.

The time has come now to return slowly, so please gather all the beautiful energy from your womb, and on the in-breath bring it up to your heart space, and on the out-breath allow it to fall down into your womb space once again. We bring this energy into your heart space, so you can feel your truth. Now on the in-breath bring this energy to your throat and on the out-breath back into your womb space. We bring this energy into your throat, so you can speak your truth. Now on the in-breath bring this energy to the top of your head, and on the out-breath allow it to flow down into your womb space again. We bring this energy to our highest selves, so we can remember and know our truth. Now, on the next in-breath, bring this energy to the top of your head and on the out-breath flow it all over your body. Allow yourself to be enveloped in this energy like in a beautiful and safe cocoon. Breathe deeply and on the next out-breath let it go. Let it dissolve and float where it needs to go. Maybe it will flow down into Mother Earth, maybe it will flow up towards the Cosmic Womb. It doesn't matter, you let go of it and stay present with your breath. Feel your breath entering and leaving your body. Slowly bring yourself back. Gently move your fingers and toes. Stretch your neck and body, and when you are ready, but only when you are ready, open your eyes.

Welcome back. I hope that you are feeling balanced and present.

Circe

Circe is a Greek witch goddess linked to magic, hunting, wild animals, education, and knowledge. Circe is known as the powerful sorceress. She was the daughter of the Sun God Helios and the Oceanid nymph Perse. She was an exquisite herbalist, and her knowledge of plants, potions, and poisons was immense. She was always associated with magic. She used her knowledge against her enemies and people who offended her, turning them into wild animals. She was skilled in the magic of transmutation, illusion, and necromancy. She lived on a mythical island Aiaia (Aeaea) with her nymph companions. She was tightly bonded with the legend of Odysseus, told in Homer's Odyssey. Odysseus visited her island on the way back from the Trojan War, and when his men became drunk and disorderly, she changed them into swines. Odysseus lived with Circe on her island, fathered sons with her, persuaded her to change his men back, and then left her on his way back to Ithaca. Another story tells of her falling in love with the sea god Glaucus, who preferred Scylla, the most beautiful of all nymphs. Feeling upset, Circe poisoned the waters where Scylla bathed, changing her into a terrifying monster. She was also mentioned in the *Argonautica*, purifying the Argonauts for the murder of Medea's brother.

We must remember that ancient Greek myths, although very important, were often told from the point of view of the patriarchy. Women were often demonised and portrayed as evil and vindictive. Gods were roaming around raping and conquering, and other women/wives took vengeance against their victims. In the 19th century, female poets began to give voice to the feminine and tell the stories from the woman's position. Circe, along with many other forgotten witches, could at last stand up for themselves. This trend spilled into the present as well. One of my favourite books is *Circe* by Madeline Miller. It is a beautiful tale weaved by Circe, banished to the island by threatened gods, and left to 'burn hot and bright in the darkness of a man's world'.

We can work with Circe in our Enchantress phase really deeply. This is the time when we are connected with our inner magic and inner transfiguration. We can shapeshift easily from archetype to archetype and draw from ourselves what we need most at this moment in time. In the Enchantress phase, we own our sexuality, our creative powers, and our bodies. The Enchantress embodies the feminine mysteries, and feminine mystique, seeing the truth of who she is and who she is becoming.

Maybe like Circe, you desire some solitude, you are beginning to let go, your reflections run deep and it's time to honour and nurture your own needs. It's time to connect to your own magic.

The Enchantress potions

Maybe like Circe, you would like to turn to the Earth and the plant wisdom. Now is the best time to listen to your intuition, to your wants and needs. Mix, cook, concoct. Be brave and daring. Connect to your inner-witch and burn the sacred fire underneath the cauldron of your feminine.

- What are you brewing?
- What are you ready to become?
- What are you still afraid of?
- What is holding you back?
- What is your power? Your gift?
- How can you tap into it now?
- What are you ready to let go of?
- What are you ready to release once and for all?

Now is the time to be who you are meant to be. Follow your interests, and your intuition. Follow your dreams. Follow the call of your soul.

Allow those little potions to help you on your way.

An Enchantress tea

- ½–1 teaspoon of Raspberry Leaf (*Rubus idaeus*)
- ¼–½ teaspoon of Rosehip (*Rosa canina* L.)

Put the herbs into a strainer, place them in your favourite cup and pour hot water over your herbs. Make sure your strainer is large enough, so your herbs can float freely releasing all their goodness into the water. Cover the cup and let it steep for 5–10 minutes. When ready, remove the plant material and compost it. Drink hot or leave to cool down and serve in a high glass with plenty of ice cubes.

If you would like to introduce more magic into your life, place your hands near the cup when the herbs are infusing and think of the intention. Infuse the herbs through your hands with the intention and then think about it again while drinking. Can you feel your inner-Circe waking up?

Raspberry leaf contains B group vitamins and vitamins C and E, as well as the minerals calcium, potassium, magnesium, and zinc. The leaves are also a source of protective plant compounds such as bioflavonoids and tannins. High in antioxidants, they support your digestive system, alleviate inflammation, and balance hormones.

Rosehips are a heart and circulatory system tonic, with powerful antioxidant and anti-inflammatory effects. They are great hormone regulators and are also nourishing, with high vitamin C. They also have aphrodisiac actions. Rose generally is emotionally uplifting, nervine, neuroprotective, nutritive, aromatic, restorative, soothing and healing for the skin (try using rosehip oil on your skin during massage or self-care and you'll see for yourself. Breasts love rosehip oil.)

DO NOT DRINK IN THE FIRST AND SECOND TRIMESTERS OF PREGNANCY, IF YOU ARE DIABETIC, CURRENTLY TAKING BLOOD THINNERS OR MEDICATION TO HELP CONTROL BLOOD PRESSURE.

Approaching the veil meditation blend

This is a blend of essential oils to use in a diffuser during meditation and any womb-connection exercises from this book. I learnt this blend from Melanie Swan of *The Sacred Womb* while I was doing my Womb Medicine Woman Training.

Into a diffuser with a little bit of water add:

- 10 drops of Frankincense Essential Oil
- 6 drops of Patchouli Essential Oil
- 4 drops of Cedarwood Essential Oil
- 1 drop of Clary Sage Essential Oil

Depending on your diffuser, plug it in the socket or light the candle underneath your oil-water mixture and enjoy.

Connecting to your inner-wisdom blend

This is a blend of essential oils to use in a diffuser during meditation and any womb-connection exercises from this book.

Into a diffuser with a little bit of water add:

- 10 drops of Lavender Essential Oil
- 7 drops of Bergamot Essential Oil

– 6 drops of Frankincense Essential Oil (*Boswellia sacra*)
– 4 drops of Frankincense Essential Oil (*Boswellia carterii*)
– 2 drops of Sandalwood Essential Oil

Depending on your diffuser, plug it in the socket or light the candle underneath your oil-water mixture and enjoy.

Sedna

Sedna is the mistress of life and death. She is the Enchantress shapeshifting into a Crone—the Wise Woman. She's the Inuit and Alaskan goddess of the sea. She provides sustenance for the body and the soul. In one version of the myth, Sedna was a beautiful young woman who was very unhappy with the suitors her father had chosen for her. Opposing her father, she is said to have married a dog. Enraged, her father took her out into the sea in his kayak and threw her into the water. When she tried to climb back in, he cut off her fingers. Angry and without hope of escaping this situation, Sedna sank to the bottom of the sea. While there, she grew a fish tail and her severed fingers became the creatures that inhabit the sea—seals, walruses, whales, dolphins, and fish. Soon she grew to love her new family and become the provider from the sea. She embraced her underworld domain and became a liminal deity. In the Inuit language, Sedna means 'Big Bad Woman'. The fishermen were afraid of this emotional, unpredictable goddess who could provide a bountiful net, or bring storms and giant waves. They did rituals in her honour to ensure she would keep providing for them.

Sedna and her seal companions were worshipped not only by the people of the far North, but North in general, also by the inhabitants of the British Isles. Some Irish families claim to be descended from the union of humans and seals. Certain female seals, known as selchies, were said to emerge every hundred years from the sea to take a human mate. They would cast off their seal skin to conceive children who, like them, could shapeshift between the worlds. Eventually, the call of the sea would prove too strong, and the selchie would return to her oceanic home. She would always provide for her human family and leave them a bountiful of fish to eat.

Sedna teaches us that we live in an abundant universe, filled with more than enough for everyone. She teaches us about polarities, about the importance of giving and receiving. The key lies in balancing the two.

Balance comes from fearlessly giving when you feel guided to and then receiving with joy and gratitude. Giving and receiving are just like breathing—both inhale and exhale are equally important.

Sedna can also help you in times when you are grieving your fertility and giving up the hope of physical motherhood. Just as her cut-off fingers became came to life, so can your projects and ideas be dressed in the cloak of form, venturing into the physical world. She teaches us that motherhood is so much more than bearing children—that we can mother our beautiful world, our ideas and, of course, most of all ourselves. She can bring solace when your bleed is approaching and when menopause starts knocking at your door.

As a queen of polarities, this beautiful sea goddess also lives in the sky. In 2003, astronomers discovered an unknown planet in the further reaches of our solar system. In a deviation from the custom of naming celestial bodies after characters from Greek and Roman mythology, they have chosen Sedna as a name for this newcomer.

As with venturing into the far reaches of our solar system and the darkest depths of the oceans, Sedna teaches us that we must delve into the dark, cold places that we fear most. Only then we can find the riches that are hidden there, and only then we will be able to find our true selves. Sedna also reminds us that even though we make mistakes, we are still worthy of love and respect. That even cast out, we can create our new reality with strength and beauty.

So, shapeshift into Sedna when you need her strength and power. Wear the colours of the sea—white, black, blue, and green. Decorate yourself with pearls, aragonite, or corals. Visit the sea to recharge your batteries, swim, drink plenty of water, and allow the beautiful feminine to envelop you with emotion and the flow. And then let go and just simply flow with all.

Beautiful cleansing bath

You'll need the following:

- Bath salts (Himalayan salt, Dead Sea bath salts, or any other organic bath salts you wish).
- Rose or Lavender Essential Oil (if your bath salts are already scented, you may skip this point, or add essential oils that are already in your salts—ex. Geranium, Fir, etc.)

- Rose petals, flowers.
- Candles.
- Coconut milk (or Oat milk).
- Intention (ex. 'I would like to purify my body and mind', 'I would like my emotions to flow freely into the water', 'I would like to connect to the frequencies of Divine Feminine', 'I would like to reconnect with my inner-most desires', 'I would like to reconnect with myself').
- Any prayers you would like to use.
- Music you would like to listen to.

1. Begin to run your bath water, as your bath begins to fill up add your bath salts (200 g is recommended).
2. Then fill a cup with Coconut (or Oat) milk and add to it 5 drops of Rose or Lavender Essential Oil. Mix it with your finger.
3. Once your bath water is full, light your candles.
4. You can decorate your bath water, your bathtub and any place that would feel nice for you in your bathroom with rose petals and flowers.
5. Before you enter the bath sit/stand facing the bath with your hands in prayer position and state your intention. You can also say out loud any prayer you have prepared for this occasion.
6. Once you are complete, pour the milk into the bath and enter the bath.
7. Enjoy your bath in silence and stillness or quietly listen to your favourite music. (You can set your intention to connect to the frequencies of Sedna, and say a prayer to her if you wish). Enjoy the scent of the oils, petals, and flowers. Allow the frequency of the water to take you on a journey within your soul.

PART 5

WISE WOMAN AND THE WISDOM REGAINED

CHAPTER 13

Menopause and the cycle remembered

Why are we so afraid of the menopause?

Menopause is a normal and healthy transition in a woman's body, but has been made into something scary and horrible, something difficult, challenging, something to dread. Something that would be better to forget about and brush under the carpet—just like menstruation, and our entire cycle stuck in a constant taboo loop. In today's culture, we worship at the fountain of youth. Youth is the ultimate goal—staying young at whatever cost. We are told that ageing is overrated and that the power belongs to those who can keep appearances of agelessness. That led us to so much fear. Fear of our bodies changing, slowing down, needing more attention and care. That also has ultimately led us to the fear of death. And what does it mean today to be an older woman in the world? Culture and civilisation are telling us this story. Sadly, we are still in the claws of patriarchy. Menopausal women are liminal women. They are at the gate of a great change. They are saying their goodbyes to the fertile years and to the monthly bleed. It's a great transition. Yet we are constantly told that menopausal women are losing it, losing their competency, relevancy, their brain. The older woman is irrelevant, she doesn't have the power, nor the status older men seem to have. Well, the time has come to tell a different story. To change this conversation. To change the entire paradigm. It is very important for us now to change our views on menopause and to prepare for it properly. It is important to understand and see how we view menopause and how we'll choose to live post-menopause. We must empower ourselves as there is a great probability that we are not going to be empowered by our culture.

The great awakening of the menopause

Menopause is not an individual occurrence. It sits firmly in the context of our life story. Story that begins at *Menarche*—our first bleed. We are going through our initiatory journey each month. It is a journey of indi-vidualisation, and maturity, and each month we have an opportunity to undergo our mini-initiation. Each month we die to ourselves and then we can be born anew. Menopause invites the big initiation forth. Initiation to which we already have a template imprinted within our being and bodies. Practising cycle awareness gives us an inside into ourselves. With this practice each month we can feel that we are coming to the end of something, and then we are opening ourselves to the birth of something new—another cycle, another wheel. When we approach menopause, we can feel deeply within that we do not need our cycles anymore, that the time has come for the big shift, and great metamor-phosis, that we are ready to step off the edge. This is a very radical initiation. One of the biggest ones in our life. So, if we all practice cycle tracking, we would be building this amazing awareness and self-care. So, we can arrive at this gate not only ready but also in touch with our health and needs. Wouldn't that be beautiful? Yet our entire lives we are told that our cycle doesn't matter. That it is not important that we do not need our bleed. We numb ourselves with hormones and by the time we get to this important transition, we are not only unprepared, but we are also unaware of our bodies, our needs and self-care practices. And when we add to it all the menopausal stories circulating in our society, no wonder that we are feeling frightened and alone. No wonder that we have no idea what is happening and what to do. And we also don't want to be the lost women, ones that don't matter, without the status and power. Simply old. Well, we don't have to be.

Menopause is a great spiritual journey. Journey where we can step into our complete and fully expanded selves. We can step fully into our power. This is the moment where we can no longer compromise anything about ourselves—the way we live, and what we think. It is a place of full alignment with our deep spiritual selves. This is the time to step into the Crone—the Wise Woman of our lives. Like our menstrual cycle is taking us month after month through this transition and phase, this life-cycle is taking us through a very similar gate. Only on a bigger scale. We have work to do to be able to step up to that level of spiritual responsibility.

The menstrual cycle is our 'direct line to ourselves'. We need all those different energies, all the archetypal powers we encounter during our cycle—this is our most important preparation for menopause. How we swim through those phases, through those transitions will give us tools to utilise when menopause will knock on our doors. When we get to know our rhythms and patterns, when we learn how to honour them, we will open ourselves to the higher levels of being. When we listen to the call of our menstruation, we can hear the hidden codes of wisdom and survival. We must stay true to that, to ourselves. We must stop cutting corners for our health. It's enough of that! We must establish proper self-care practices and utilise them month after month, allowing the time of the Dark Feminine to become a time of true renewal and re-birth. We are guided from within, so the time has come to listen to this guidance—journal, write it down, and think about it. Find time.

Please think for a moment about the energies of your menstrual cycle. We start in the darkness, expanding into the fullness of light at ovulation and then contracting once more inwards, towards the depths of ourselves and the surrounding Dark Feminine. The energies of our life-cycle are just the same. We begin in the darkness of the womb, then expand through childhood, young adulthood, and maturity—Maiden, Lover, Mother, Enchantress, reaching the gates of the Wise Woman. We are young and strong, then waxing into the fullness of our potential, but after that the energy is beginning to wane, just like the moon. With the decrease of strength comes tiredness. It seems quite obvious. Yet, when we reach the gates of menopause and we are exhausted, we are surprised. This is another gift our society gave us. The society that doesn't allow slowing down, taking a break and simply being. Often at the time of the beginning of menopause, women are still in full-time jobs, children may have not yet left the house, pets need our attention, and housework needs to be done—no wonder that we are arriving at the gates of the menopause exhausted. The problem is that we won't have the opportunity to recharge.

This transition takes a lot from the body and mind. And as there is no honouring menopause as the sacred event that is going to happen, there is no sense of preparing ourselves in a way that is sufficient and honouring to ourselves. So, we reach this gate imagining that we can cope with it somehow—we have coped with life pretty well so far. Sadly, we are met with the greatest surprise—it doesn't work that way. At menopause, you are coming to the end of the great cycle in your life. This is one of the most vulnerable moments, the time when we have the least energy, and least stamina. This is the nature of this process. You are going through death and that will bring certain emptiness, certain loss. You need to allow that death to happen, just like you allowed the end of each cycle in your life. At the gates of the menopause, we are faced with grief. The great grief of the fertility passing, the grief of losing our cycle, of losing our bleed. From now on we are not going to be able to fertilise the earth with our blood, it is going to stay within. In the beautiful cauldron of our womb, we are going to stir this potent elixir for our own purposes. Where do you think the wisdom of the Crone comes from? It comes from within her, from the depth of her retained blood. So welcome that grief and allow yourself enough time to process what has passed. Process all that you are losing in this transition. But at the same time prepare yourself for this amazing metamorphosis and open your mind and body to the wisdom you have cultivated your entire life.

There is no way around it. But don't despair. Although not the easiest of times in your life, it doesn't have to be as horrible and difficult as patriarchy is making us believe it could be. You need to meet yourself, your needs, and your desires. And by following the path of your cycle, you may already have a huge knowledge of those, and you may have self-care practices already put in place. If not, you must think about it now. You must remember.

Alexandra Pope and Sjanie Hugo Wurlitzer call them our sacred tasks. Tasks we all need to undertake to help ourselves through this Mother of Transitions. You need to rest more. Life is busy, I know, but without rest you will burn yourself to ashes. Introduce 1% of change and build it up 1% at a time. This is not optional. You must find time and spaciousness for nourishing yourself on all sorts of levels. You won't pour from the empty, and without rest and taking care of yourself you will become empty sooner than you think. It really is all about nourishment. How do you nourish your soul and your body? Give yourself some time to dream—dream into your soul. Dream your new reality into being. Put boundaries into place. Make conscious decisions about what you are able and cannot do. If someone asks you to do something—pause before you answer. Take stock. Don't answer straight ahead. Say instead—can I check with you tomorrow; I need to check my calendar. Write in your calendar—*Sacred time for me!* And treat this time as the most sacred thing in the entire world. Do not override it with other commitments. This sacred time is non-negotiable. Think about your diet. Are you nourishing your body enough? Remember, you won't pour from the empty. What is good quality food that gives you pleasure? Find willingness in yourself to take care of yourself. This is what we must teach our children. We can teach by example. Do not forget about pleasure itself. Find the pleasures in your life. What brings you pleasure? Pleasure for your body, for your mind, for your soul. Reach for it, grab it with both hands.

Make a clear intention—how would you like to experience menopause? How would you like to live post-menopause? This is something not many people are talking about, but there is so much healing happening during this phase. Can you welcome the deepening wisdom? How do you want this experience to unravel? How do you want to experience yourself post-menopause? How do you want to be seen? What would you like to do? How do you want to live? Write it all down. Intent for it to happen the way you would like it to. Look at older women out there in the world. Fabulous older women, role models.

I would like to be an older woman living well. Living fully in my power. Doing my thing. Loudly, without fear nor shame. I would like to feel my own authority. Not shadowed by the authority of someone else. I would like to hold the meaning of my life in my hands. To feel the empowering fierceness of my own power. Even if others would try to dismiss me, I will never dismiss myself. I would like to fully embrace my womanhood with all its shades and textures. And I am welcoming the Old Crone, the Wise Woman of what is yet to come. I embrace her fully. Will you?

CHAPTER 14

Welcoming the Wise Woman

Autumn

Autumn is such a beautiful season. It marks the transition from summer to winter. The duration of daylight is becoming noticeably shorter, and the temperatures cool down considerably. Day length decreases and the length of the night stretches immensely taking us all deeply within. The striking change in the colour of the leaves shows us their readiness and preparation to shed. We can learn so much from the trees. They don't fight with the seasons. Instead, they welcome the change and are letting go. Leaf by leaf, colour after colour, down to the ground in the great transition, preparation, and retreat. Into death and darkness, waiting for the turn of the wheel to take them back into the light, re-birth, and renewal. They are waiting patiently, standing stoically, retreating within. And with the trees all the rest of nature is preparing for the winter to come. Animals gather food in their forest's larders, preparing themselves for times of absence and shortage, and some for the time of hibernation. Those who don't hibernate but can't stand the cold are gathering strength and coming together before the great departure. The rest are preparing for what is to come. Autumn is the time of the last harvest. Fruit, vegetables, and grain are still ripe at the onset of the season, and we can feel the gratefulness in our bodies— Thanksgiving time.

There is the feeling of gratitude and plenty, but also the melancholy for the time gone and the one to come. The possibilities and opportunities of summer are truly gone, and the chill and change are on the horizon. Skies turn grey, and the descending darkness becomes palatable in the air. People also react to that change by turning inwards, into the depths of their own bodies and souls. The maturity of the world has reached its peak and the only thing following is brought forward by Lady Death. Autumn is very strongly associated with Halloween feast and All Souls Day. The celebration of life and death, with the time to honour the ancestors and to invite their wisdom into our hearts and homes.

Autumn is usually portrayed as a mature woman surrounded by apples and vine leaves, holding the grapes. She often holds the Cornucopia filled with fruit and abundance given from the land. In the polarity of life autumn is at once a symbol of plenty, ripening, harvest, celebration, and abundance, as well as decay, decline, old age, and even death.

Crone, Sage, or Wise Woman?

It's all in the name. The potential to feel empowered or disempowered. The ability to lead or to stand at the end of the queue with your head down. The power of the word is immense, even if we pretend to play it down. In stories we tell ourselves, the Crone is often seen as something to be feared. She is ugly, evil, old, and petrifying. She is a representation of death and its mysteries, and from times immemorial, things that are unknown were always feared. But if we think about it for a moment, we can begin to tell ourselves a different story. The word Crone is derived from the old word for crown. It suggests the wisdom emanating from the head like a halo. That woman is the queen. Her own childbearing years are in the past, and now she is the wisdom keeper, seer, and healer—the Sage and Wise Woman. She is a midwife, whose knowledge should be sought out to help guide others during life's journey and transitions. She is the wisdom personified. By connecting to our inner-Crone we begin to listen deeply within. We are preparing for the winter and the wintering, closing the cycle, and honouring our bodies. By connecting to our inner-Crone, we at the same time are connecting to the Sage and Wise Woman, as they are always coming together. They are one and the same.

Wisdom of the Crone

The Crone invites us to look within, to slow down and regroup. The energies have been coming back to us since the Enchantress began her reign, and now they are pouring within with the doubled force. Within your body, the barriers between the conscious, and subconscious are beginning to wither, and you are able to open your awareness to the consciousness of your body. The veil between the worlds begins to thin. If you listen to this phase and won't try to suppress it, you will begin to feel a sense of acceptance and you will feel yourself being part of the greater All. The creative energies are changing too. They are no longer inspirational but are becoming more visionary. Your Seer is coming forth and if you welcome her with an open mind and heart, with curiosity, she can show you places that can change you forever. This phase brings you closer to the phase of stillness and gestation. This phase shows you the steps of descent into your inner-most self. Your body responds to it too. You start to have less strength and energy, you may begin to feel heavier, more swollen, and you may need more rest and sleep.

The outside world becomes less important and sometimes even annoying. Social things become unnecessary. You can hear the call of your inner world. Your patience level decreases, and your inner-critic takes over. The critic is sharp-tongued, as all the filters are coming down. Intellectual processes often slow down, but the emotional ones well up to the surface. Sexual energies are present on an entirely different level and the need to express the depth of love and romance and being witnessed and mirrored by the partner become very strong. Sex becomes the expression of the deepest, sensual, and spiritual love between you and the other. It could also unravel that deep, sensual, and spiritual love for yourself. This phase is the end of the outwardly dynamic energies of your cycle. It is preparing you for the end. This ending can bring a sense of loss, if the new and inner qualities are not recognised. But approaching the end can also help you with cutting ties with everything that holds you back. It is preparing the fertile cave of your womb, enabling the seeds of new ideas to germinate there during menstruation, so they can grow forth when the new cycle comes.

Can you see how much wisdom the Sage/Crone can bring us if we listen deeply within? If we begin to prepare for wintering, honouring our bodies, honouring the Grandmother that lives in every one of us, honouring the Wise Woman, honouring the Midwife.

During our inner autumn, everything comes into sharp focus and often it is a time of review. Ask yourself these questions:

- What have I lost during this cycle?
- What do I need to let go of?
- What do I need to grieve for?
- What is hiding in the shadows?
- What do I need to release to bring more balance into my life?
- How did this cycle show me how well I'm communicating my own boundaries?
- How well have I been honouring the boundaries of others?

If you allow it, this phase of your cycle can become a storytelling time. Not dominated by the Hag living in the house in the middle of the rotten woods and eating children, but by a Wise Woman sitting at the fire with a circle of women and weaving wisdom from within. The more we listen and share, the more we remember; and the wisdom of the stories can carry us through the darkness. This is true Womb Shamanism.

We must make sure that we allow winter to happen, that we allow her to come and cover us in silence, in darkness, and in time that flows in a totally different way. We must allow our bodies to get ready for rest, introspection, and slowness. We must stop acting like autumn and winter are not happening. Katherine May wrote in the 'Wintering': 'In winter, you're never more than a few steps from darkness'. It is so very important to remember that and to prepare our bodies and minds. Autumn is the time of preparation—preparation for the winter. Humans, especially us women, have forgotten how to properly prepare, and how to rest. We must remember it as darkness could be a double-edged sword. It could be a time of rest, rejuvenation, seership, and bliss, but it could also be the time of terrifying shadows taking over.

The beauty and the challenge of pre-menstruum is that your shadow awakens. All the things you've neglected throughout this cycle, all the feelings you've pushed to the sides, all the historical woundings and generational traumas that have been relegated to the unconscious, can now break free and demand recognition. Only here do you have the power to hold that tension, to recognise it, to feel it fully within and allow it to be. And by allowing it to be you are allowing the healing process to commence. And all those shadows are not pretty—some are terrifying, some are very sad. And holding it in being is a very difficult task. If you decide against it and try to push it even deeper out of the consciousness of your body, this is when this phase will bite back. With difficulties, frustrations, anger, outbursts, hormonal fluctuations, difficulties with sleep, and nightmares—your body will show you that there is a process to behold. Your pre-menstrual reactivity, rage, self-sabotage, and self-rejection is a crying for help from the little girl within, whose needs haven't been met. Presence and self-holding are an act of self-love that will allow you to soften into your wisdom. The little, forgotten girl will be able to, with great pleasure sit down on her grandmother's lap listening to the weave of her stories. You have both, the little girl, and the grandmother within, so allow yourself to be fully illuminated, conscious and present. You can now truly face yourself and all your aspects, all archetypes.

During this phase, all your questions, even the difficult ones, will be answered truthfully and deeply. The inner-critic is awake and ready, and the filters are down. You will think as it is and you will say as it is, without taking any prisoners. You can really get to know yourself in your inner autumn. You will discover where your edges are, and you will be able to create boundaries that will suit you, not the others. Your inner senses are heightened, and you will become more and more sensitive to what is happening around you and within you. The noises will be louder, the smells stronger, and you will just know things. Always listen to that inner knowing. If you won't acknowledge your inner-critic and won't befriend her in your inner autumn, she will turn against you with self-sabotage, self-hate, and many other destructive behaviours.

For just a little while you become a truth-sayer. Your tolerance to let things go will be much smaller and your fuse much shorter. What you say may not be received with gratitude, but it will be important. You will become insightful and will be able to see both sides of every situation. But if you don't recognise the depth of this phase, you may easily be persuaded to jump from one side of the story to the other.

Many women find that their creativity is very heightened at this phase. You can almost become a pure channel and birth whatever needs to come into this world. You can embody the Midwife archetype and be present for the unspoken and the unmanifested. This is the power of deep embodiment. Through your body you can cross the border to the other side and see, feel, or hear the patterns that create everything. You can channel this inner Shamaness with ease and inner strength. I like to imagine myself in my inner autumn as a wild old woman. One, who doesn't care how she looks like, as she doesn't have to impress anyone anymore. One, with wild hair, long flowing skirts, or naked, dancing around the fire. One, who 'runs with the wolves'. One who doesn't care what the world would think, as she got rid of the shame bounding her to the common standards of society. I imagine myself free in the depths of true freedom. I can feel the creation flowing out of my body, and I midwife it into being, with patience and wisdom. I am myself and I am All. If embraced, this is a truly majestic and a wonderful place to be. If rejected, this is a place of a great pain, misery, and struggle (PMS).

The Wise Woman is not afraid of her uniqueness. She doesn't need to fit in, and she knows it. She cherishes that knowledge. She can be kind, but at the same time she won't be polite, nor socialised. She will be true—true to herself and her values. This is a part of your initiatory journey—a journey to find yourself. Every cycle you are standing in front of the great changing and flowing, you look into the mirror of your archetypes, and you are getting ready. You are getting to know yourself and preparing yourself to arrive at the gate of the Mega Change, the menopause, and by the time you get there, you will hopefully discover who you are becoming, and you will be able to embrace it fully. By opening yourself to yourself and your needs, you will be able to learn all about compassion and that in turn will open you to become compassionate towards others. Only in this way, you will be able to feel a deep belonging to life.

But the secret lies also in the flow and in letting go. You cannot always rule. You must allow yourself to be vulnerable, tired, and fragile. Do you remember, in this season your energy is draining out and is gathering inside your womb, so it can flow with your beautiful bleed. You must not expect yourself to stay on top of things. This is the best moment to practice the art of surrender. Give up on the outside world, go deeply within and flow with whatever you'll meet there. Shake hands with the grandmother and sit with her at the sacred fire. Share wisdom and listen to stories. The world won't end because you won't participate in it for a moment. If you preserve your strength and replenish it, you will be able to flow with bliss during your bleed. If you go against yourself, and use all your strength, over-exhausting and overworking yourself, your bleed will bring you pain, inability and despair. And the winter that comes after will be truly barren.

The Crone will show you exactly where you are, even if you don't want to see it. She will show you what needs to change, what needs your attention, and what you've been doing great. You will get feedback on everything—your health, sleep, stress levels, emotions, unresolved issues, projects, relationships. You will get feedback on your life. You can choose to fight it and remain deaf to the wisdom hidden within. Or you can accept this feedback and stay present and kind to yourself while receiving it. The Crone will call you to use all the self-care practices you can master. Listen to her, you will never regret it. Go slowly, surrender, and be emotional, there is nothing wrong with that. Be self-aware but don't allow self-sabotaging and self-destruction to play the first violines. They will only come if you will deafen yourself to the call of your Wise Woman. Without self-compassion and self-kindness, autumn can bring you destructive storms that will havoc your life. Remember, you are returning to yourself, to your cave of wisdom, strength, and power. This is a reason to celebrate, not dread and hide. This is a reason to answer the call and to embrace the wild woman within.

In our pre-menstrual phase as well as in the physical season of autumn, we are welcoming the darkness within and without, and the time of All Souls and Halloween. This is the time of meeting the ancestors. The Wise Woman knows how to travel between the worlds. How to move the energy over and through the gates. She can connect, commune, and learn from her ancestors, from the teachers, and from the Earth Keepers. She is a sacred traveller, a seer with the power of the oracle. This is the first gate that you will cross to Dreamworld. The second one will welcome you at the onset of your bleed—the Gate of Deepening and the Great Beyond. Prepare yourself to receive these teachings. Start dreaming. You won't dream if you won't allow yourself to slow down and to rest. You won't hear if you won't allow yourself to be open and to listen. You won't commune nor communicate with the other side if you are too busy running around like a headless chicken, burning the candle at both ends. If you go against your body and the season, nightmares will try to get your attention and teach it in a less pleasant way. The information will be coming across, as the veil between the worlds becomes thinner and the knowledge is passing through. It depends entirely on you what type of communication it will be. If you open your Wise Woman's eyes, your inner grandmother will take over and she will lead you across the bridge to gain wisdom beyond beliefs. Why fight this beautiful gift? Open yourself to receive it fully. Flow with the power of seership. This is the place where you can receive the most intimate answers to the most intimate questions. This is the place of deep knowing.

If you are still struggling in your premenstruum, there may be a deeply held trauma from the time before your birth. Both inner autumn and inner winter are an amazing mirror of that time in our past. If you still have a mother, ask her about the conception and pregnancy. If you don't or prefer not to, journey to the past and discover it for yourself. What happened during the seeding of your soul? Was the womb you had chosen for your first home hospitable or hostile? It all reveals itself in our menstrual cycle, as our cycle is the mirror to our soul, our true self. Was your arrival waited for and cherished, or was it dreaded and filled with misery? We carry within us many generational traumas, and we pass them on to our children without even knowing. How was your grandmother when she was pregnant with your mother? Was she happy and supported? How was her birth experience? All those questions are vital for our well-being.

In the West, we count our days from the moment of birth, and we forget that this baby was already here for the previous months— listening, experiencing, loving, and fearing. What was your gestational time filled with? Loving or fearing? If you are able to connect to your grandmother. Listen to her stories. Ask questions. Don't waste that time anymore. If you can, allow your inner grandmother to meet with your grandmother and see how this relationship can develop. Maybe from this point in your cycle you will be able to understand your granny and her decisions better. Maybe from this point you will be able to forgive her. In today's world, many women suffer from endometriosis and adenomyosis. Both conditions are causing scar tissue. When you think about it, how many emotional and physical scar tissues are we holding within? Unhealed trauma is kept and passed from grandmother to granddaughter. We know now that we keep trauma in our bones and tissues. How much of this trauma can be accommodated before we start to experience the physical symptoms? Because believe me, physical symptoms will come. I know it so well from my own experience and from the experience of many women I have been honoured to work with.

It's not an easy path and it won't change anything overnight, but my personal experiences with adenomyosis taught me that by resolving the past traumas I could help myself with present pain. Not only that. I've journeyed many generations back, witnessing the trauma of my grandmothers and my aunts. It gave me a huge understanding of what is happening to my body today and why. It allowed me to see, witness and forgive, but also find more self-compassion and self-love. It allowed me to become part of my female ancestry line and claim this position fully. And my sacred task is to try and work through as much trauma as possible, so then the next generation doesn't have to carry so much. Again, it is not an easy task, but one worth undertaking. So be curious, observe, allow yourself the flow of the mysteries, step back from the outside world into your inner-most depths, and ask questions, journal, journey, rest, process, and flow. This is the sacred task of the feminine.

If you don't bleed anymore, welcome the Wise Woman fully into your life. Allow her to show you the paths beyond, allow her to open your true eye. With this eye see the past and the future. Soften into your changing body, without judgement and expectations of youth. Welcome the *Change*, become the *Change*. Susan Weed said in her beautiful book *New Menopausal Years*: 'now you are holding your wise blood inside and stir it in your own cauldron, you will nourish yourself, your Kundalini, your serpent power, and find yourself, at 60, passionately sexual with all of life'. It doesn't sound like a curse of a Hag, does it? It sounds lovely and juicy. It sounds nourishing and enriching, magical even. To be able to keep the blood within the cauldron of our wombs, to nourish, to feed the serpent, to rise to the knowing. No wonder patriarchy is so frightened of this time and that knowledge. Knowledge that has been feared for many thousands of years. Don't you think that the time has come to reclaim it for ourselves, for our daughters and granddaughters? The time has come to embrace the Wise Woman within fully and allow her to speak the words of wisdom through our mouths and *Yonis*. So, open your ears. Listen. Speak up. Flow.

This is the time of autumn, of wisdom embodied. This is the time of descent. The goddess is leaving the world, and the heavens and descends into the underworld. She goes there to be challenged, to meet up with her sister, lose virginity and maidenhood, to be changed. To shed her old skin, her old self and be re-born as someone new. And with this newness come more attributes and more power, as by now she is not only the goddess of heavens and the world, but she is also the goddess of the underworld. She has come a full circle, and she has become All.

CHAPTER 15

Dancing with goddesses: the Wise Woman

Innana

Innana is an ancient Mesopotamian goddess of love, beauty, war, and fertility. She is associated with sex, divine law, and political power. She was originally worshipped in Sumer under the name Innana, and later by the Akkadians, Babylonians and Assyrians under the name Ishtar. First, the heavenly goddess of the sky, and one of the Earth and Nature, creator of life, she became the creator of death and re-birth when she descended into the land of her sister Ereshkigal.

One day, Innana decided to visit her sister, Ereshkigal, in the underworld, to attend the funeral of Ereshkigal's husband. Her sister decided to teach her a lesson, and as she passed through each of the Seven Gates of the Underworld, she had to leave behind one article of clothing or jewellery (all that made her powerful and mighty queen), so that when she reached her destination she would be completely stripped of her worldly power. When Ereshkigal saw her sister coming naked in the purity of her being, she set upon her and killed her. She then hung her corpse on a meat hook and left it there to rot in the sun. Before she left her palace, Innana instructed her maid and helper, Ninshubur, to get help if she didn't return within three days. After three days had gone, Ninshubur went to the god of wisdom, Enki, for aid. With a clever plan, they help Innana to come back to life and escape. Before she left, Innana was told that she would have to find somebody to take her place in the underworld. She decided to send her husband, Dumuzi, as he had not mourned her when she was gone. But because Dumuzi was missed so much by his sister, Gestinanna, and his mother, Ninsu, Dumuzi and his sister arranged to trade places with each other every six months, so that each would only have to spend half of the year in the underworld.

Innana teaches us about the importance and inevitability of the descent. For whatever reason from time to time each of us will descend into the depths of darkness and death, a place so hopeless that we lose faith in any possibility of rising again. Yet Innana gives us back hope. She teaches us that death is followed by a re-birth and the life-cycle continues. Not like we knew it before, because it is impossible. With each re-birth, we are wiser for our experiences and lives before. She is teaching us about the journey we all must undertake to reach our wholeness. Innana is filled with light, but she must appear before her darker half—her sister, she must die and return to life to be able to combine and balance the light with the darkness. She descends into darkness, sheds her former self, is confronted with the shadow, with the death of who she was, and is re-birthed as a completely different self—this time fully aware.

So do we, women, every month at the end of our cycle descend into the end of that cycle, into its death. And in the darkness of our void, in seeming nothingness, we have a chance to be re-born, to enter the new cycle and new possibilities. And each time we are wiser for all the experiences of past cycles, for each of the deaths and re-births we undertook. And if we do it consciously, each time we have an opportunity to become more complete, to become whole.

It also happens when we stand in front of the great change of menopause. This is the greatest descent a woman can attempt. When we face the Crone, our fears, and our shadow, we can learn who we are now and who we are becoming. We can find and embody our wholeness in an entirely new way. Sometimes all it takes is a leap of faith so we can take the first step into darkness of ourselves. We would have to strip into our naked core and look deeply within our corpses. Only by embracing the death of who we were, we can allow ourselves to be re-born anew.

The descend meditation

Please sit comfortably, with your hands on your lap and your feet firmly on the ground and close your eyes. Take a deep breath in and out to arrive at this point in time, at this practice. Sigh out on the out-breath and let go of the day, of everything you have done so far, and all that you are still planning to do. You are taking time out for yourself. This is your time and your practice.

Please breathe naturally in and out. Don't force it. Notice your breath coming in and out of your nostrils. The cold air is coming in, it warms up inside your body and the warm air is flowing out. Gently and naturally, in and out. Feel how your body is relaxing.

Your feet are letting go and with each gentle in-breath, the relaxation is going up your body. When you breathe out your calves and shins are relaxing, then your knees and thighs. Breathe this lovely energy up. Your hips are relaxing, and your pelvis, your abdomen, and your waist. Relaxation is coming higher with every single breath. Now your ribcage is relaxing, your breasts, and your shoulders. Relaxation is going down your arms and into the palms of your hands. Your hands are heavy and fully relaxed. Your throat is relaxing, your jaw, your tongue is relaxed in your mouth. Your nose is relaxing, your eyeballs and eyes, and the lines on your forehead are straightening and relaxing. Your head is fully relaxed. Your body is heavy, your breath is slow, and you are fully relaxed now.

Just breathe gently in and out

Now on the out-breath, I would like you to imagine strong roots growing from your feet and anchoring you in the ground. The roots are strong and mighty. On each in-breath lovely nutrition and strength flow straight from Mother Earth into your body. On each gentle in-breath, this nutrition is flowing up to the top of your head nurturing all the organs and tissues in your body. And then on each out-breath, it's going down your body, to your feet and then through your feet into the roots and back into Mother Earth. And on each out-breath, I would like to invite you to send all your love and gratitude back to Mother Earth. Beautiful communication between your body and the body of our Mother. You are well nurtured, you are grounded, you are safe. Let's take three deep breaths in and out through our roots to nourish our bodies.

On the next in-breath, I would like to invite you to take the energy all the way up, to the top of your head and pause there. Breathe deeply in and out and imagine that you can see a beautiful staircase leading from the top of your head right down into your womb. There are 12 steps, and we are going to walk them down into your womb space while counting backwards. Stand on the 12th step, breathe in and on the out-breath, you are going to start walking down. Are you ready?

Take a breath in and out and step down—11, 10; you are going down and down; 9, 8, you are passing a narrow corridor of your throat; 7, you are going down; 6, 5, you are passing right by your heart, a mighty drum; 4, 3, down and down; 2, 1. You are down at the gates of your womb. Open the gates and walk in. You are in your womb space now. Look around. What does this space look like today? How does it feel today? Look around ... Feel ... Become ... Breathe deeply into your womb space.

Let the life-giving force of your breath enter your womb space. As you see, feel, or sense your womb space notice that she is very dark. Let this dark womb be like the dark earth. And here in the womb is a cave and a place of great comfort. Place of solace and rest. Place of quiet and the dark. Notice any fears or resistance that come up from going into these depths of darkness. Notice them without judgement, but with curiosity and compassion. And if you are willing, also notice the comfort of being here, relaxation and peace. And if you are willing you can call upon the archetype of Innana, of the Crone, you can call in those who know how to go into this dark place, and ask them to guide you, to help you see what is there in the shadows. Some aspects of yourself that were pushed into this depth, that are not feeding you. And aspect of your soul that has cut itself from you. Some part of you that was stuck in the underworld. Part of you that you have forgotten about. Or maybe was ashamed of it. See that part and allow yourself to embrace it. This part is still safe right here, within you. Allow your subconscious to show you the part that would like to rise now. A part that has had enough of being hidden in the shadows. The part of yourself that you have been missing, that you haven't had access to for a very long time.

Breathe deeply. Bring your awareness to what it is and imagine it as a seed. And if you are willing take this seed in the dark and plant it deeply within your womb space. And conjure the energy from the Great Mother, through your roots, from the part of you that is the Mother, and allow the little seed to be enveloped in safety, nourishment and love of germination. Breathe into it. Deep into yourself. As you exhale, feel the life energy rising, flowing, and spreading through the darkness. Activating, germinating, fertilising the seed within you. And allow this seed to flow with this sacred energy. Allow your womb to show you what this seed is. How is it going to grow and what is it going to become? Just breathe into your womb space. Into the darkness. See this seed is beginning to grow. Within it is the part of you that is returning. Welcome that part back. Breathe into that part. See it clearly. Say quietly: 'Welcome home'. Find the Mother within you and the Wise Woman and welcome this part back to your body, to your consciousness, to your energetic field. Welcome back, my darling. Welcome back. Breathe deeply.

Now allow the light to enter your womb space. Feel her shining with life-giving light. Feel your seed rooted deeply. Feel this part of you fully back. Completely merged back with you. And in this moment in time, feel yourself whole once again. Breathe deeply. Allow yourself some time to process everything that has happened. Come back to the presence within your womb. Thank your womb for this beautiful gift, for being re-born. Smile inwards and outwards.

Now the time has come to return. You are ready to leave your womb space. On your in-breath gather the energy of your womb, so you can take it with you. Now walk back to your womb's gate. Walk through the gate and close it behind you. This is your womb space. Your sacred space of power and you can return here whenever you wish. Now the time has come to walk back. You can see in front of you 12 steps ascending. Approach the lowest step. With each breath in you are going to step up the steps, you are going to walk up. Are you ready?

1, 2, 3, higher and higher; 4, you are passing by your heart, a mighty drum; 5, 6, with each in-breath you are going up; 7, you are passing a narrow corridor of your throat; 8, 9, 10, 11, 12. You are back at the top of your head. Take a deep breath in and on the out-breath flow this beautiful womb energy that you have brought up with you all over your body. Envelop yourself in your womb energy like in a cocoon. You are safe, you are grounded, you are loved.

Gently start to bring yourself back. Move your body, wriggle your fingers and toes, move your neck and when you are ready open your eyes. Gently notice your surroundings. Look up and down, left, and right. Feel yourself fully embodied and present. Drink some water. Journal. Welcome back, my darling. Welcome back.

Persephone

Persephone is the Greek goddess of spring, and the Queen of the Underworld. She is the queen of the cycles of life, death, and healing. She was the daughter of Demeter and Zeus. The story of her descent to the underworld and her eternally recurring return to the earth has been a central religious theme. She goes through a transformation only death can grant you. As Kore, she is the goddess of seeds, flowers, and corn. She is a Maiden, beautiful in her innocence, in her spring. Desired and kidnapped by Hades, she transforms, matures through the presence of death and her time in the underworld, and discovers her new purpose. She becomes the Wise Woman, the healer, the midwife, and the goddess of the life–death cycle.

Persephone's abduction by Hades has several versions and is mentioned by Hesiod in his *Theogony* and in the *Homeric Hymn to Demeter*. Zeus, Persephone's father, was a conspirator in her abduction, and permits Hades to carry the young goddess off to his realm. Hades was disheartened by previous rejections by Demeter of Hermes and Apollo, when they were courting the young goddess, so instead he went straight to his brother. Overprotective Demeter deemed all unworthy of her daughter and took her far from other gods to keep her safe. When Persephone was picking flowers with her companions, Hades burst through a cleft in the earth and took her in his chariot to the underworld. Demeter mourned the loss of her daughter and searched for her all over the Earth with the help of Hekate's torches. She relinquished her blessing on the land, making it barren, until she got her daughter back. Zeus sent Hermes to Hades to demand the goddess be released to appease her mother, but before she left, Persephone ate some pomegranate seeds. It meant she couldn't fully return to her mother and could only do it only for part of the year. The other part she must spend with her husband in the underworld. Persephone entered the underworld as a naïve girl but returned to Earth as its queen.

The ancient stories told from the patriarchal point of view refer to the first encounter of Persephone and Hades as a rape and abduction. She is portrayed as a victim of the circumstance and the power play of her parents—a chauvinistic father, who just gives her away, and an overprotective mother, who wants to hide her and keep her for herself. Neither Zeus nor Demeter consider what the young goddess wants. This is how I saw this story for a very long time. But now, I believe differently.

I think Persephone chose Hades and she allowed herself to eat the pomegranate seeds to stay in the underworld. She remained fluid in the face of change and adapted to new circumstances. She became transformation itself. Persephone's willingness to return to the underworld and then to the world of the living allows her to work through times of change and undergo the mysteries of life and death. Only in this way, can she grow. She accepted the crown on her head and gave up the archetype of the sacred Maiden. From the hidden girl, she became the sovereign queen. I absolutely love the book of poems *Great Goddesses* by Nikita Gill. I love it because it shows myths from a very feminine perspective. Persephone is not a victim here; she is not naïve; and she is conscious of her polarised nature. She is not defined by the abduction or by the male dominance. Each story is flowing, and the meaning sleeps underneath everything we know. In the poem 'Demeter to Hades (A Mother's Fury)', Demeter says:

> I will give this union no blessings.
> Not when even your presence
> will harm my fae daughter.
> She is a child of flora,
> of fauna, of fruit,
> too gentle for your hell.

This is how I always saw Kore. A being so delicate she would not survive in the presence of the god. But Persephone has within the strength of the Divine Feminine. She will not only survive his presence but will also match his strength and power. She is a worthy and desired companion. In a beautiful poem, 'Persephone to Demeter', Persephone says:

> But, Mama, he found me. He saw me
> nourish this beast in the woods,
> fell in love with the part of me that
> no one else could, promised me a land where
> I could be a queen and not another version of you ...
> Mama, you gave birth to a girl
> who knows her own mind. He didn't snatch me
> and take me to hell. I went there because
> I wanted a queendom destined to be mine.

I think it's quite refreshing to look at Persephone as a queen in her own right, destined to rule over hell, alongside her demonic husband.

Persephone is the great guide when you need help with the courage to face life's challenges. For when you find yourself torn between two powers, when you need to face your shadow and look it in the eye. She will give you strength when you are facing the unknown. Persephone embodies the true ownership of self. She accepts the change and flows with it, adapting with fluidity. She praises the time of the darkness and rest and understands the burden of being always in full bloom. To avoid getting burned we must find in ourselves space to descend into the darkness and rest, to retreat within as Persephone does.

Dancing with your shadow

For this practice, you would need your favourite piece of music, a darkened room, candlelight, or a light that will enable you to see your shadow on the wall, a journal, and comfortable clothing. You can also do this practice naked if you wish.

Get yourself and your space ready. Darken your room, light your candle or the lamp and place it in such a way so it's behind you and you can clearly see your shadow on one of your walls. Start your music and stand facing your shadow. Breathe deeply. Close your eyes and centre yourself. Feel your feet on the ground, feel yourself grounded, and embodied. Breathe deeply into all corners of your body. Feel your breath filling you up with life-giving energy. Feel your breath filling you with relaxation and peace. Breathe deeply and find your presence. Presence in this room, in your body, in your life. Can you feel it?

Open your eyes and look at your shadow. This is an integral part of you. A part you cannot escape or hide from. It's always there. We were programmed to believe that the shadow is scary, even evil, and that we don't need it. That goodness lives only in the light. But the truth is that shadow is an integral part of our life. A very important part. This shadow is going to tell you the story of your strength and power, of your beauty and perseverance. Look at your shadow now. Feel her presence. Now imagine, sense, or feel that your shadow is swaying gently in the rhythm of your music. Allow your body to follow the movements of your shadow. In this order—first your shadow, then your body. It may be challenging at the beginning but trust the process and flow with it. Follow the movement of your shadow and dance with her.

Allow yourself to be lost in the trust that she will lead you where you need to go. Dance with your shadow. Immerse yourself fully in this experience. Allow all the emotions that want to surface to come to the surface of your being. Do not stop anything from flowing. Follow your shadow on this beautiful intimate journey. What is she showing you? What hurts? What pain is coming to the surface? Where? What feels pleasurable, good? Allow your thoughts to leave your head and just concentrate on following your shadow and feeling within your body, whatever wants to come. Become the feeling, fully embodied. Descend into your shadow world. Dance with your shadow.

Spend some time in this practice if you feel comfortable. At some point, you may notice that your shadow is slowing down. Follow her and allow your body to slow down. Slower and slower, until both of you meet in stillness. Thank your shadow for all her lessons and close your eyes. Breathe deeply. Feel yourself coming back from this journey. Feel yourself being present in your body, in your room. Feel yourself in full control of your body. With your eyes closed turn around from your shadow. When you open them look around your room, but don't look at your shadow. Right now, you are going to leave your shadow behind you, and you are facing your future. Remember that she is always there; she will support you whenever you need her. Gently and lovingly for yourself look around your room. Allow yourself to return fully to your body and into your space. When you are ready, take your journal and describe your experience. Describe your dance with the shadow. What did she show you? What did she teach you? What has changed within and without?

Please drink some water and if you still don't feel fully back, eat some grounding food—banana, some nuts, root vegetables, soup.

Welcome back to the union with your shadow. Welcome back home to the whole you.

Baba Yaga

I grew up hearing stories of Baba Yaga. In the story I grew up with she used to live in a house on a chicken leg, and she ate children. She was evil and she needed to be outsmarted to survive. But who really is this scary and mysterious old lady?

The story of Baba Yaga came to the world from Slavic tradition. 'Baba' means an 'old woman' or 'grandmother' in most Slavic languages.

She is described as a terrifying, ugly old witch who presides over our fate and destiny by deciding whether to listen to our requests and make them happen or devour us. She lives in the middle of the forest in a log cabin perched on the chicken foot/feet. The house can change around so that Baba Yaga can view every angle of the forest at any time. Not an ordinary witch, she doesn't travel on a broom, but instead she uses a mortar to fly in, using the pestle as a rudder. Her broom, which is typically made of silver birch, trails behind, clearing the racks of her whereabouts. In some stories she is a single being herself, in some she is a part of the trio of sisters of the same name. Although very often she comes as a representation of the wicked witch, she is much more complex than that. She is cunning, clever, and mostly a hindrance, but can be helpful, and when you look at this from that perspective she is the first feminist in the folktales.

Baba Yaga doesn't care how she looks, what others think, or what she does. She doesn't feel the need to explain herself to anyone and she does as she pleases. By eating children, she is standing in strong opposition to the nurturing mother and is showing that women can be more complex than what patriarchy wants us to believe in. She lives by her own magical terms and doesn't allow anyone to create rules for her. Baba Yaga is a shamanic trickster. She crosses the boundaries of what we are comfortable with and what a description of an older woman should be like. She shows us that true freedom lies beyond the borders of social norms and that darkness within is as important a teacher as an inner light. She may be hidden in the woods, but her house allows her a wonderful vantage point. She is always present and always watching.

Baba Yaga is showing us the importance of every aspect of femininity, every drop of womanhood, and she brings with her great lessons. She unveils harsh truths and allows us to see what is holding us back. She brings freedom and magic. In our culture an older woman doesn't mean much, she has no power, and in a society that worships youth we try at whatever cost to prevent the Crone from coming. In ancient societies, older women were the keepers of mysteries, wisdom, and tradition for the entire community. They had status and respect. They understood the mysteries of life and death, they were healers and midwives that could help the souls onto and from this world.

Patriarchy taught us to fear Baba Yaga, to be afraid and to avoid the fearsome, strong, independent feminine. We have been taught that we can see the world from the perspective of the victim, of the weaker gender. But Baba Yaga shows us that this is not true. That each of us holds wild feminine within. Feminine that doesn't care about social norms, that is not afraid of the darkness of the woods. Feminine that is strong and powerful.

Baba Yaga is showing us that we can be self-sufficient and independent. She teaches us that we can take ownership of our actions, and that we are strong enough to abandon the role of victimhood. We can be scary and terrifying, and we are also a force to be reckoned with. She is showing us that our happiness cannot be defined and be dependent on others and our opinions can be validated only by us and us alone. Baba Yaga's lesson is to embrace the cycles of life fully with curiosity and gratitude. She says to us—hold on to the past, to being a victim, to being a child, fight the flow—and I will devour you! Take ownership of your own independence and self-sufficiency—and I will help you to grow. Baba Yaga's lessons are the hard ones. She bestows on us the gift of change and loss. She will destroy any denial and ignorance that is stopping us from truly knowing ourselves and that prevents the death process. New beginnings cannot be birthed without the death of the old and Baba Yaga is here to prepare us for the next round. In nature life, death and re-birth are present constantly, and the cycle tracking is helping us to refer to and find ourselves in this constant flow and change. All of nature—the cycles of days and nights, the waxing and waning of the moon, the journey of the sun, the turning of the seasons in the wheel of the year—all our life is reflected in our cycle. To interact with Baba Yaga is to interact with death herself. She is a truly magical entity based on the earliest idea of the Wise Woman. To connect with her aspect within you is to connect with the healing wisdom of Crone. And through her death rites, she will ease us into the void and allow us to prepare ourselves for the birth of the new cycle that will arrive with the first drop of our blood.

Questions to journal with

- What is keeping you from relying on yourself?
- How can you tap into your confidence more?
- What can help you to trust more in your own decisions?
- What does darkness mean to you?
- Who is Crone for you? How can you embody her more?
- What does it mean to be a Wise Woman?
- What does it mean to you to be truly independent?

– How can you prepare yourself for the dark season?
– What brings you pleasure at this time in your cycle?
– Is it really that important what others think? Why?

Wise Woman mandala

Many people say that our most creative time is during our summer/ovulation. I personally find that although my creativity is super heightened during that season, it is also coming strongly to the surface during autumn. My descent creativity is different than the summer one. It's much more oracular and with many layers of inner depth. I feel drawn within, into the coming darkness of the void, into a place where everything is possible, and all can happen. Through my inner vision, I traverse time and space and while waiting for my bleed to come, I can tap into the powers beyond my body and my imagination. This is the best time to seek your own truth. To switch your thinking mind off and allow your spirit to soar. This is why I would like to invite you to explore the Wise Woman mandala.

In Hindu and Buddhist symbology, a mandala is a circular figure representing the universe. It represents the spiritual journey, weaving like a spiral from its outside layers to the inner core—and every layer is filled with meaning. In Jungian psychology, a mandala as a symbol in a dream represents a dreamer's search for completeness and self-unity. Mandala can represent the map of the universe and can enable us to delve deeper into the hidden realms of the unconscious. Mandalas are present in every religion and tradition of the world bearing different names but similar meanings.

I would like to invite you to translate the reality of your cycle into a pattern. Into the map of your personal universe. As you are standing now at the gates of the void, look back and notice the lessons, meaning and symbolism of your cycle. Don't overthink it, remember, we are in Baba Yaga's realm. Connect to your wild inner-wisdom, let go of expectations and create your map.

You would need a quiet place to sit, a candle and matches, your favourite music if you wish, a piece of paper with a circle drawn on it (as large or as little as you wish—if your mandala will grow during creating you can always draw a bigger circle around the first one), and art materials—crayons, pastels, pens, pencils, paint, pages from the glossy magazines (for the collage mandala)—you are the creatrix, chose the medium that speaks to you the most.

To create your mandala, first prepare your sacred space. Light the candle and sit quietly in contemplation. Using breath, will and imagination connect to your womb. Ground yourself and spend some time connecting and listening to the messages from your womb. Set your intention: 'My intention is to create the mandala of my current cycle'; 'My intention is to draw a map of my cycle'; 'My intention is to translate the reality of my cycle into a pattern of this mandala'; or whatever intention you feel yourself called to. When you have set your intention and when you feel ready take the colours and begin your mandala. Don't think about it at all, just be present and do what comes. Allow yourself to give in to this process entirely. Chanel the colours, shapes, symbols—don't think about the meaning behind them, not yet—this is your place to connect to the wild feminine, the feminine that is pregnant with creativity and power, and direct it all into the piece of paper in front of you. Remember, Baba Yaga doesn't ask for permission, and you don't need to either. Be in the moment and let it flow, let it become. Allow your entire body to flow with it. If you feel like you want to stop painting and start dancing—do it! If you feel the noise rising through your body—let it rise and release it without fear or shame but in total pleasure. If you feel the pleasure building in your *Yoni*, don't shy away from it but embrace it wholeheartedly, release it, let it flow, and join with the creative energies of the universe. If you feel slowness and meditative energy embrace you, allow it to happen—slow down and meditate. And then when you are ready come back to your mandala. You don't need to rush, you are not in a hurry—take your time, be present with whatever is rising, and witness yourself and this moment of your cycle. Fully embody the creatrix that you are.

When you feel complete, stop drawing and look at your mandala. What can you see? What does it mean to you? What was revealed? Don't use your logical mind to read your map—use the eyes of your womb, your feminine wisdom. You know the meaning already; it is woven into the fabric of your being—access it and allow the translation to come freely. Whatever comes embrace it. This is you, and you are perfect as you are. This is you, and you are as powerful as you are. This is the map of your cycle, with its beauty, meanings, and lessons—approach it with kindness, love, and compassion. This is the art of your life—recognise and cherish it.

And most of all have fun connecting to the maps of your life and your cycle.

CHAPTER 16

The Elemental Woman

We are all born as elemental children of the universe. We are all connected through the beautiful universal web of life. Each of us originated from the same source. From the powerful, elemental ancestors of Air, Fire, Water, and Earth. Our bodies are elemental and composed of water—blood, sweat, tears, birthing fluids; earth—flesh of our beautiful bodies, our bones; fire—energy, and air—breath. Through archetypal knowledge, we are given the lessons and the opportunities that will enable us to change. To flow with the Great Mystery of Life. We are all the Elemental Women, and we are ready to remember this once again.

There is much to be written about the elements and their importance in our everyday lives, and this will be the topic of my next book—*Womb Shamanism—the Elemental Woman*. But for now, let me mention the importance of elements in our menstrual cycle.

To understand it deeply we really must open ourselves to the wisdom of being the elemental children of the universe, the divine creations of our ancestors—the human and the elemental ones. And divine we are, as the spirit is embodied within us. We are the spirit made flesh. And when we look at the elements, we must remember that just like us, they have both a spiritual and material aspect at the same time.

Only through this knowledge and remembrance, we can alchemise our lives. Only through this alchemy, we can allow the change in, to grow, develop, flourish and to become the better versions of ourselves. To become who we were meant to be.

When looking at elements, the seasons, and our menstrual cycle, it is very easy to fall victim to generalisation and schematisation. I've seen others teaching and rigidly holding the schematics of Spring—Air, Summer—Fire, Autumn—Water, and Winter—Earth. There is little space here for movement, flow, and shift. The only possibility in this diagram is to connect the nearest elements to one another, so the transition between spring and summer will hold air and fire, the transition between summer and autumn will hold fire and water, etc. But what about the Indian summer or all the other in between seasons that we are holding within? Don't they have the right to elemental power? Well, they do, and they have. We must remember—we are the Elemental Women, not the Diagram Women. The feminine flows and cannot be locked in ridged frames.

Our body is like a cauldron that mixes all the elements together and in our wombs the flesh, the blood, the breath, and the energy come together in a beautiful alchemical miracle. The physicality and the spirit joined together in the sacred union. They infuse one another, mixing and brewing and when the shift happens and the right season turns, the best representative for us in this moment will surface through. And it may be different for you and me, depending on where we are on our life journey—but it may also be the same. The elements are filled with manifestation. Some of the elemental manifestations are quite natural and obvious. The stability of the Earth, the transformative powers of the Fire, the fluidity of Water and the expansiveness of Air, they are all dancing within us, looking for our own, individual balance. The art of elemental knowledge is to dive deeply into each and every one of them to feel how we embody each one in different aspects of our lives. And here also we can call on archetypes for help.

The Earth Woman

She is like the force of Mother Earth herself. She is stable and nourishing, supporting all around her. She is selfless, reliable, and practical. She is grounded and solid. She is filled with her bodily presence, aware of her form and edges. She is the foundation of life, the mother, growth, and fertility. She is feminine and receptive. She is strong and filled with sustenance. She is free through roaming the Earth and can find freedom through limitations, as she can easily overturn them into positive traits. She is relentless, practical, secure, accepting and patient. She is a great companion and has strong craftsmanship. The Earth Woman's negative qualities can be heaviness, dullness, boredom, stagnation, resignation, lack of initiation, or leaving everything to others.

Earth Woman loves her curves, thick hair, and smooth skin. She has endless vitality. She can make love all night and then get up in the morning and conquer the world. She doesn't make on-the-spot decisions, she may not be very adventurous, but she likes to consider all the options. But once committed, there is not much that can stop her. Life for her is like making love—slow, steady, and deep. She loves spending time in nature and is not afraid to get a little dirty. She has a sharp eye for detail and wants things just the way she wants them.

The Water Woman

The Water Woman flows with life. She enjoys life to the fullest— sensuality, art, good food, beauty, and the delights of living in the world. She allows herself to be expressed through living in the world. She has so many hidden depths, secrets and mysteries hidden beneath her shimmering surface. She is always showing new forms and facets of herself. She can adapt to new situations easily. Her vitality and creativity cannot be bound. She is connected to her feminine consciousness and the subconscious. She loves the moon and feels fed and nurtured by her light. She loves the night and is not afraid of the dark. She can look into the mirror and see all the depths of herself, and she has the ability to show in that mirror the depths of others. She is receptive, dreaming, and perceptive. She has great imagination, intuition, and the ability to dream her world into being. She holds depth, prophecy and knowledge and can deeply connect to all her feelings. In her negative aspect, she can be spineless and give into the victimhood mentality. She can struggle with dependence, vagueness and lack of interest and commitment.

The Water Woman flows with emotions. Her inner world is incredibly vivid and colourful. This inner life, the dreams, and the imagination can become more real to her than the material world. She is highly sensual, incredibly artistic, and creative. She relies on her feelings and allows them to guide her through life. She is romantic, often tearful (the water is always near the surface) and affected by everything deeply. She needs to feel intimately connected to her partner and to life in general. She seeks pleasure through all her being.

The Fire Woman

The Fire Woman burns with passion, enthusiasm, and excitement for life. She is radiant, and always shining. She thrives on adventure and generally is very intense in everything she does. Her temper can be frightening, but at the same time she has warmth and generosity. She is a leader, courageous, confident, and unshakeable. Her willpower is strong. She is mysterious and filled with true purpose. Her mind is lively with wit and ideas. She sees sharply and is aware of everything that is happening around her. She is magical and the magic in her will never be embarrassed by the rational mind, as her mind is passionate and sharp as well. She has force in her character and strength in her purpose and whatever she does will make a long-lasting impression. In her negative aspect, she can be cunning, deceitful, superficial, impractical, and blinded by her own ideas and intelligence. She can be dictatorial, bad-tempered, erratic, chaotic, over-imposing, and destructive.

She has a lot of heat in her body, and a need for constant movement. She likes to move fast, makes quick decisions, and sometimes acts impulsively. She feels everything intensely and can be very reactive. Everything can be stormy and intense, but the storms pass quickly. She looks for passion in love and in life. She looks for excitement. She is bored by softness, but the danger is always appealing. When she commits to something, she is all in and she expects the same from others. She prefers love and life to be lived and experienced fast and sometimes rough. In the heat of her body and the drumming of her heart, she can find happiness and release.

The Air Woman

The Air Woman is light and graceful. Her vision and inner vision are unstoppable, spreading in all directions. She loves freedom above all. She is open to possibilities and explorations. Nothing can hold her down for long. She needs to fly. She loves to connect and talk to others. Her words flow with ease, and she is filled with clarity, poetry, and expression. She is a peacemaker and brings harmony through communication. She is filled with incredible ideas and inspiration. Her intellect is incredible, and her life is filled with soul. She is inspirational. She is often scientific, light, and clear-headed. Inquisitive and problem-solving. She is rational and this rationality can tip her into the negative aspects. She can then overuse dry intellect and can be harsh, absent-minded, confused, and uncertain. She can become detached, overly logical, penetrating, and cruel.

The Air Woman's hair is thin and fine, and her skin tends to get dry. She walks through life with her head in the clouds. She is bursting with creativity and curiosity. But she may have trouble finishing things as her attention moves very quickly to something new. She is in constant movement in her body and mind. She falls in love easily and with her whole heart. But if her heart gets broken, it doesn't take long to mend it and move on. She is filled with gentle touch, tenderness and heart connection with everything and everyone.

The Earth Woman, Water Woman, Fire Woman, and Air Woman all live combined in your body and soul. Some are more active some are more dormant, nevertheless they are all within you. So is their archetypal knowledge—all contained within. Ready to surface at any point. Surfacing right now. Stop for a second and look deeply within. What does your Earth Woman look like? What does your Water Woman need? What is your Fire Woman telling you? What is your Air Woman trying to show you? In this moment in time, in this moment in your cycle, which one is coming to the surface with her teaching and wisdom? Which one is more dominant? Which one you are not able to see/feel at all? It is all-important. It all brings messages from your inner world, from your wellness and from the point where you know if your needs are being met. Which of them is trying to get your attention? To be noticed, seen, understood? Are they whispering to you, talking loudly, or maybe shouting for your attention already? What is happening within? You have learnt how to live with your menstrual cycle and by now you can observe it with the keen hawk's eyes. Where are you in your cycle today? What is going on in your body? In your mind? What element dominates here? Is it in its positive or negative aspect? How can you help yourself to feel better, or to maintain the feelings you are enjoying right now? Look to the wisdom of the dominant energy and to the wisdom of the lack of energy you cannot feel at all. Maybe another element needs to be invited in.

So, if you find yourself amid the fire-filled summer, look deeply within. How is your water doing? How is your earth? Maybe you will find that your Earth element is drowning in a muddy bog, so you can call on the power of the scorching heat to dry it up, so you can ground yourself properly and feel earthed once again. Or maybe the fire element is too strong for you to cope with right now and you can call in the cooling power of the wind, the support of the earth and the refreshing ability of your inner rain. Or maybe your fire is just right, so you can flow with passion and creativity and put yourself out there, into the world. You are holding this power within. You are the Elemental Woman.

Allow yourself to discover which element is surfacing more often than the other when you are in your Maiden phase. Which one is coming forth in the Lover or Mother phase? Which one is pulled forth by the Enchantress, and which one is called by the Crone? Is every cycle the same? How does it change when you travel through the sun cycle? Which elements come forth during spring, summer, autumn and winter? What is happening with the moon then? Do you feel fire rising at full moon, or does the moon call in the waters of your being? Don't let anyone tell you what is right and what is wrong, what you should be feeling. Notice yourself. What is happening *within you*? And when you notice it all, allow the wisdom and the healing energies of the elements, phases, and all the archetypes to flow through your body, through your mind, through your soul. Embrace them fully. Embody them. Don't be afraid. Be in the flow—you are the daughter of the Sacred Feminine. You are the spirit embodied. You are amazing. You are so strong and resourceful. And the answers to all the questions of the universe are already embedded within your body.

As the elements have both spiritual and material aspects, you can call forth either one of them if you feel unbalanced in your body or soul. I've worked with these elements in my Bardic and Shamanic training, and I found them extremely useful in the cycle tracking and womb-work as well. If you would like to work with the elements individually, get to know them and connect with both spiritual and material aspects of them, you could follow some of these exercises.

Working with the Earth element

Go for a walk in nature.
  Do some gardening.
  Meditate with crystals.

Sit underneath the tree with your back to the tree trunk and feel yourself grounded in the earth. Feel yourself becoming one with the tree, supported by the earth, one with all.

Walk barefoot on the soil, grass, and stones—feel it all underneath your body. Become that feeling, that connection.

Lie down on the earth (try doing it naked). Place your arms and legs in the most comfortable position. Your womb connecting and touching the fertile soil of Mother Earth. Breathe, be, feel. Absorb the earth's forces and give back your love and gratitude. Feel her power, stability, safety, and 'groundness' entering your body, your womb. Feel the energies of Mother Earth balancing the Earth element within you. Breathe deeply.

Journal with some questions I found in the book *Practical Ceremony* written by my wonderful friend, Pia Tohveri, and some of the questions I go to when I need more earth in my life.

- 'How does Mother Earth show her strength to you?'
- 'Can you feel fully grounded and let go of stuck beliefs?'
- 'What are your roots telling you?'
- How are your roots feeling?
- 'Are you feeling nourished or starving in your soul?'
- What secrets is Mother Earth sharing with you right now?
- What does the Earth element within you need right now?
- Can you recognise the song of your Earth element? Can you sing it out loud?

Working with the Water element

Go for a swim.

Take a long, relaxing bath.

Take a shower with the intention of the falling water connecting to and awakening your Water element within.

Go for a walk near the river.

Go to the seaside. Put your feet/submerge yourself fully in the sea and feel the power of the water.

Work with your menstrual blood.

Fill a bowl/chalice with water, and sit in meditation gazing into the water. What can you see? What comes forth?

Listen to the pulse of your own blood. Can you feel your own rhythm? Can you move to this pulse?

If you cannot physically get to the seaside/river, then you can connect with water through meditation. Intention, will, and imagination are the keys to this type of work. Lie down or sit comfortably. Visualise yourself floating on the water; swimming or diving in the depths of water; diving down and rising to the surface. You can visualise yourself as a water being, made entirely out of water. How does it feel like? How do you flow as a water being?

Journal with some water questions.

– 'Are your emotions flowing freely?'
– 'When do you feel the most balanced?'
– 'Is your natural flow blocked, and if, what can you do to release it?'
– How do you feel about crying? What does crying mean to you?
– What secrets is Mother Sea sharing with you right now?
– Can you hear the voice of your blood? What does it say?
– Is the water in your life flowing or is it still? Is it full of crushing waves and stormy pools?
– What does the Water element within you need right now?
– Can you recognise the song of your Water element? Can you sing it out loud?

Working with the Fire element

Light a candle and meditate by looking into the flame. In stillness merge yourself with the flame.

Light a bonfire and dance around it.

If it is safe, jump over the fire. (You can use your candle and jump over it as well).

Imagine yourself as a fire being, entirely made up of fire. How does it feel like? What does your fire dance look like?

In meditation, visualise yourself as travelling to the sun. Imagine yourself landing on our life-bringing star. What does it look like? What can you see? Can you charge your body and your soul with the fire that surrounds you? Imagine lying in the sun and soaking in the fiery energy. Where does this energy go within you? Which parts of you need it the most?

In meditation, visualise yourself as walking through/into the fire. Imagine this fire to be as big or as small as you wish, so you can feel comfortable and safe. Imagine yourself standing within and burning. But there is no pain, no fear, only transformation. In your meditation, who is coming out of the fire when your old self burned away? Who is this new creation? What did you transform into?

On a sunny day sit or lie down comfortably in the sun. Allow the warmth to spread all over your body. Allow it to soak in, the light and the warmth, through the layer of your skin, through the veins, organs, and bones, into the core of you. Open yourself fully to receive both—the light and the warmth.

Open your *Yoni* to the sunlight. Allow the warmth of the sun to linger on your vulva. If you feel it is right for you at this moment, imagine it entering you and filling you with the beautiful and healing masculine energy of the sun. Feel the warmth inside you. Allow this energy to be awakened within your body.

Make passionate love to yourself or to your partner.

Journal with some fire questions.

- 'What is your passion?'
- How does the fire speak to you?
- What is stopping your transformation?
- 'How can you keep connecting to the Fire element?'
- What parts from within are you ready to burn?
- What does your fire look like? Does it burn brightly or is it struggling?
- Draw your fire. Dance the fire dance. What can you do to bring more creativity into your life?
- What secrets is the Fire sharing with you right now?
- What does the Fire element within you need right now?
- Can you recognise the song of your Fire element? Can you sing it out loud?

Working with the Air element

Concentrate and connect to your breath. Take each in-breath and out-breath mindfully.

In meditation, allow your breath to travel all over your body. Allow it to reach the places that you usually don't breathe into—breathe into your feet, knees, and hands. Breathe into each organ in your body and bring there this beautiful life-giving force.

Breathe into your heart and then into your womb.

In meditation, imagine yourself flying. How does it feel like? Are you flying as yourself or has your body changed somehow? If it has changed, who are you now?

In meditation, imagine yourself as a being made entirely from air. How does it feel to be in the air? How does it feel to be Air?

In meditation, imagine yourself as a consciousness only. You have no body to stop or limit you. You are pure consciousness. How does it feel? What is happening to you now?

Go for a walk on a windy day. Feel the wind dancing around your body. Allow it to penetrate you.

When outside notice the breeze or wind moving around. What direction is it coming from? How does it make you feel?

Fly a kite.

Journal with some air questions.

- 'How can you work with the air energy to nurture your heart space?'
- How can you work with air energy to nurture your soul?
- 'How does the air element communicate with you?'
- How is the airflow in your life right now? Is it a gentle breath, a loving breeze, or a violent storm? How can you work with what is happening?
- Dance the air dance and describe your experiences.
- Can you breathe freely and fully? If not, what is stopping you?
- What secrets is the Wind sharing with you right now?
- What secrets is your Breath sharing with you right now?
- What does the air element within you need right now?
- Can you recognise the song of your air element? Can you sing/ whistle it out loud?

You are the Elemental Woman. You are surrounded by the elements, and you are holding their power within—every day, always. It really is up to you to notice which element is surfacing in every stage of your cycle and draw in the medicine from it. Do not let anyone tell you how you should be feeling or which of the elements should be present in this or that phase. Allow the elements themselves to come forth and speak with you, speak to you. Open yourself to their lessons and wisdom. Invite them in, manifest them, embody them, and release them allowing the free space to be filled with the new one—the best one for your changing phase. And in this beautiful dance of Water, Air, Fire and

Earth, find your rhythm. Find your elemental dance and allow yourself to fully release into it. To let go of your expectations and just simply flow—the flow of the Sacred Feminine embodied within your soul and DNA. You already are the Elemental Woman. You already are holding this power within. Remember, be, flow.

Dear fellow traveller, thank you for walking with me along the path of the women's mysteries. I truly hope that it has been for you a journey of self-discovery and self-love. It surely has been for me. When I started writing this book, I had no idea what powerful medicine it would bring to my life. How much change and revelation I will discover myself. Following the cycles of our beautiful planet, the sun, the moon, and my own body allowed me to open myself to the true meaning of the embodiment. To experience life truly through my body, to accept who I am and consciously reach for who I am meant to become, for who I am becoming. When you look at cycle tracking from a shamanic perspective you become an embodiment of Paradise on Earth. And you can understand that nobody is excluded from that embodiment, and that death is just a doorway from one stage to the other. The wisdom of our Medicine Wheel is immense and can help us to consciously face all the obstacles and trials that life, our families, and society are throwing our way. It's not enough to promise yourself that you will try, that you will observe, that you know that already and that you can be kinder to yourself and others. The secret lies in actively engaging the archetypal energies that can change the paradigm of our values and actions.

Following Carl Jung's description, we can understand that archetypes are the 'forms in the psyche which seem to be present always and everywhere'. The archetypes described in this book are very ancient and have guided human thought and experience for a very long time. Archetypes are embedded in mythology and are woven into our everyday lives. They represent the underlying forces of nature and through them, we can find empowerment and re-find our way back home to ourselves. We are all carrying within our personal myths and often we think it's only us in the entire world who is suffering so profoundly or can love so deeply. The teaching of the archetypes shows us that the entire human race is able to embody all of them. Although each of us is the heroine of our own personal journey, we can draw from the wisdom of the generations past and the stories they have left behind. Despite the wisdom of the old stories, it is greatly important and helpful in our lives to remember that the time has come to create our own and new mythology. It is important to understand and embody what your Maiden feels like; what your Lover desires; what your Mother needs; what your Enchantress represent and what your Crone is whispering in the depth of night. And maybe by following your cycle you will discover entirely new archetypes rising. How wonderful! Embrace them, their wisdom, and their teachings, because this is what you need in your life at this moment in time. This is what is important to You. So, you can embody your life fully and truly. Only by breaking free from worn-out beliefs, and from the dictatorship of others trying to tell us what we should think and feel, we can change our lives and our destinies. And our cycle, like the great Medicine Wheel that it is, can be our vehicle to implement those changes and observations.

To reclaim our power, and to reclaim ourselves. Our cycle provides us with a great map of tackling the challenges of everyday life and of transformation that we are embodying daily. No one can do this work for you, but that also doesn't mean you have to walk alone. I hope that this book has proven to you that you are in a great company of wise women discovering their bodies, cycles, and the meaning of their lives. Preparing the journey for the new generations and easing the pain of the generations past. And by mastering the lessons of each archetype you can transform your life and embody it fully. You can embody the wisdom of your menstrual cycle and step into the wisdom of your sacred spiral, deepening your knowledge and skills at every turn and in each new cycle. And through this process embody the magic, power, and strength of your womanhood.

Thank you for travelling with me, and for your time and application. May we meet again.

BIBLIOGRAPHY

Ahmed, A.M., Iat the Milk Goddess in Ancient Egyptian Theology, *Journal of the General Union of Arab Archaeologists*, Volume 2, Issue 1, Article 2.

Ann, M., Meyers Imel, D., *Goddesses in World Mythology*, Oxford University Press, 1995.

Bashford, S., *You Are a Goddess: Working With the Sacred Feminine to Awaken, Heal and Transform*, Hay House, 2018.

Buckley, T., Gottlieb, A., *Blood Magic: The Anthropology of Menstruation*, University of California Press, 1988.

Butler, S., *Moon Power: Lunar Rituals for Connecting With Your Inner Goddess*, Fair Winds Press, 2017.

Cancer Research Trust, New Zealand, Stories, Dr Erin Macaulay, The Placenta: That Tissue That Nourishes New Life May Also Save Lives (www.cancerresearchtrustnz.org.nz).

Gill, N., *Great Goddesses: Life Lessons From Myths and Monsters*, Ebury Press, 2019.

Gordon, S., *Popularna encyklopedia mitow I legend*, Amber, 1998.

Gray, M., *Red Moon: Understanding and Using the Creative, Sexual, and Spiritual Gifts of the Menstrual Cycle*, Dancing Eve, 2009.

Guerber, H.A., *Myths of the Norsemen: From the Eddas and Sagas*, George G. Harrap & Company, 1922.

Hendrickson-Jack, L., *The Fifth Vital Sign: Master Your Cycles and Optimize Your Fertility*, Fertility Friday Publishing Inc., 2019.

Jung, C., The Concept of the Collective Unconscious, in *The Portable Jung*, ed. Joseph Campbell, Viking Penguin, 1971.

Miller, M., *Circe*, Bloomsbury Publishing, 2019.

Pearce, L.H., *Burning Woman*, Womancraft Publishing, 2016.

Pearce, L.H., *Moon Time: Harness The Ever-Changing Energy of Your Menstrual Cycle*, Womancraft Publishing, 2nd edition, 2015.

Peters, F.K., *Reclaim Your Dark Goddess: The Alchemy of Transformation*, Rockpool, Summer Hill, 2022.

Pinkola Estes, C., *Women Who Run With the Wolves: Contacting the Power of the Wild Woman*, Rider, 2008.

Pope, A., Hugo Wurlitzer, S., *Wild Power: Discover the Magic of Your Menstrual Cycle and Awaken the Feminine Path to Power*, Hay House, 2017.

Pope, A., Hugo Wurlitzer, S., *Wise Power: Discover the Liberating Power of Menopause*, Hay House, 2022.

Reardon, S., Ancient Virus May Be Protecting the Human Placenta, *Science*, 27 October 2022.

Room, A., *Botanical Medicine for Women's Health*, Second ed., Elsevier, 2017.

Shuttle, P., Redgrove, P., *The Wise Wound: Menstruation and Everywoman*, Marion Books, 2019.

Star Wolf, L., *Shamanic Breathwork: The Nature of Change*, Brave Healer Productions, 2022.

The Order of Bards, *Ovates and Druids*, Bardic Companion.

Tohveri, P., *Practical Ceremony: A Creative Journey With the Elements*, Pia Tohveri, 2022.

Tresidder, J., *Symbole i ich znaczenie: ilustrowany przewodnik zawierajacy ponad 1000 symboli wraz z objasnieniem ich tradycyjnego i wspolczesnego znaczenia*, Horyzont, 2001.

van Wyk, B.-E., Wink, M., *Medicinal Plants of the World. An Illustrated Scientific Guide to Important Medicinal Plants and Their Uses*, Timber Press, 2004.

Varulker, R., *Moon Woman: Feminine Lunar Journey*, ARN. China Ltd, 2020.

Virtue, D., *Goddess Guidance Oracle Cards*, Hay House, 2002.

Waldherr, K., *Goddess Inspiration Oracle Guide*, Llewellyn Publications, 2007.

Weed, S., *New Menopausal Years: The Wise Woman Way*, Ash Tree Publishing, 2002.

Woodfield S., *Dark Goddess Craft: A Journey Through the Heart of Transformation*, Llewellyn Publications, 2021.

www.aleteia.org (Why is the Virgin Mary Feeding St. Bernard with Milk?)

USEFUL LINKS

1. Using Reiki, Zero Balancing & Doula services to find your inner strength (primetherapy.co.uk)
2. Yes Yes Yes. Natural, Certified Organic Intimacy Product Experts—YES (www.yesyesyes.org/)
3. Welcome to your Doorway Home | Spiral Song | Womb Medicine Woman (spiral-song.com)
4. Come home to your true nature. | The Sacred Womb®
5. Womb-Work with Jamie Wiggins M.A. (www.jamiewiggins.org)

www.ingramcontent.com/pod-product-compliance
Lightning Source LLC
Chambersburg PA
CBHW071741270326
41928CB00013B/2758